*Lives Worth Living*

Women's experience of chronic illness

Veronica Marris

An Imprint of HarperCollins*Publishers*

Pandora
An Imprint of HarperCollins*Publishers*
77–85 Fulham Palace Road
Hammersmith, London W6 8JB
1160 Battery Street
San Francisco, California 94111–1213

Published by Pandora 1996
10 9 8 7 6 5 4 3 2 1

© Veronica Marris 1996

Veronica Marris asserts the moral right to
be identified as the author of this work

A catalogue record for this book
is available from the British Library

ISBN 0 04 440938 9

Printed in Great Britain by
Caledonian International Book Manufacturing Ltd, Glasgow, G64

All rights reserved. No part of this publication may be
reproduced, stored in a retrieval system, or transmitted,
in any form or by any means, electronic, mechanical,
photocopying, recording or otherwise, without the prior
permission of the publishers.

In memory of Pam Muttram,
1959 – 1992,
with love and thanks.

# Contents

| | |
|---|---|
| *Acknowledgements* | vii |
| *Introduction* | 1 |
| 1. Feeling Different: Isolation, Invisibility and Identity | 9 |
| 2. Feeling Useful: Work, Roles and Contributing to Society | 48 |
| 3. Strange Attitudes: Coping with People Coping with Us | 72 |
| 4. Not a Real Woman?: Love, Sex and Families | 101 |
| 5. Biting the Hand that Feeds Us: Dealing with the Doctors | 140 |
| 6. Passing the Buck: Who Is to Blame for Illness? | 183 |
| *References* | 210 |
| *Biographies of the Women Interviewed* | 215 |
| *Glossary of Illnesses and Medical Conditions* | 221 |
| *Index* | 226 |

# *Acknowledgements*

Many thanks for providing contacts, information, resources or encouragement go to the Department of Applied Community Studies at Manchester Metropolitan University, Greater London Association of Disabled People, Parent-Ability, Women's Health (previously Women's Health and Reproductive Rights Information Centre), Positively Women, Maternity Alliance, Greater Manchester Coalition of Disabled People, Manchester Disability Forum and North Manchester Women's Health Team.

Also many thanks to those who commented on the text or offered advice at various stages, including Folasade Agbalaya, Sue Backhouse, Hilary Brooke, Julia Cameron, Lynda Carroll, Ruth Collett, Brenda Ellis, Hilary Ford, Rohina Ghafoor, Lorraine Gradwell, Alison Hennegan, Kate Hill, Beth Humphries, Michael Kerrigan, Caroline McGrath, Jane Morris and Linda Pepper.

There are many, many other people from whom I have learned much and gained much encouragement and support, including all the women I have met through the Women and Diabetes Network; staff and members of Central Manchester Community Health Council; colleagues at the Self-Help Resource Centre; Sara Dunn at Pandora; friends Jill, Marion, Lis, Sean, Julie, Debbie, Jackie, Kate, Mark, Mary and Heather; cousins Claire and Alison; all of my family, especially Phil and Jessica.

Finally, and most important of all, my thanks to the

women who shared with me their time, thoughts and experiences and whose lives form the substance of this book.

I am indebted to Reed Books for permission to reprint the extract on page 18 from *Spell # 7* by Ntozake Shange, Methuen, Reed Books, London, 1985 (in association with the Women's Playhouse Trust).

# Introduction

I began working on this book because I looked in vain for one like it after being diagnosed with insulin-dependent diabetes at the age of 27. Books on diabetes seemed to offer little information for or about women like myself, while books about women included little about illness, let alone about diabetes. The invisibility of my experience frustrated and depressed me and, had I not had a close friend who had developed diabetes a few years earlier, I would have felt very alone.

Together with two other diabetic women, we started a small self-help group. After a while we advertised the group in *Balance*, the magazine of the British Diabetic Association, and received a flood of letters from women who wrote of their loneliness and misery as they struggled with eating disorders, the menstrual cycle and pregnancy, with little help from uncomprehending or downright hostile diabetes clinics. During the seven years since then, I have met many other women with diabetes who have talked about these and other experiences; but most of all about the problems caused by the hidden nature of our illness and by the labels and rules imposed on us by others.

So, like many books about women, this is about the invisibility of our lives; it also deals with our struggle – as women, disabled people and patients within the National Health Service (NHS) – to retain control over our bodies and our lives.

While it all started with my own experience of diabetes, three years of advice work with self-help and women's groups left me feeling that many concerns and problems must be common to women with a range of illnesses or medical conditions. Increasingly, I have come to identify myself as disabled; not an identity I find easy or straightforward. As a member of disabled people's organizations, I have felt at times slightly fraudulent because I have not experienced the oppression faced by those more visibly disabled or those who become disabled early in life. I have also felt marginalized or out of place, as there seemed no space in which to voice my feelings about being a disabled woman, in particular a woman with an illness.

For me, the enormous importance of the disabled people's movement is that, in this era of post-feminist, post-socialist, post-everything individualism, fostered both by the right and by some alternative philosophies, it is an area of politics where people still talk about changing the world rather than adapting individuals to fit into it. Belonging to the disabled people's movement has changed my perspective on politics and on life itself in fundamental and important ways, but it has also left me still feeling isolated in coming to terms with illness.

I think the main or only thing that unites disabled people, perhaps more than any other oppressed group, is an environment of oppression. Many of us have nothing in common with each other other than that we fall outside the very narrow category of what counts as 'normal'. There is a world of difference between someone born deaf but completely healthy, a wheelchair-user injured in childhood, and someone with cancer or heart disease. We experience oppression itself very differently according to when and how we become disabled, the extent to which our disability is obvious to other people, and other important factors such as our race, class, gender or age.

With other diabetic women I can complain (and joke) about injections, blood tests or feeling ill. Many disabled people who are not ill, however, do not want these negative feelings aired any more than do non-disabled people. American writer and disability activist, Anne Finger, writes in *Past Due* about speaking in public of the horrors of surgery in childhood, only to hear one woman say that she would have killed a child of hers rather than have them go through that:

> My heart stops ... It is my old fear come true: That if you talk about the pain, people will say, see, it isn't worth it. You would be better off dead.[1]

There are powerful reasons for us to emphasize the good aspects of life with disability and to deny the bad; not only in order to create a strong and positive disability culture, but also to protect our lives. We are constantly threatened by the non-disabled world which fears 'catching' our impairments and resents sharing resources with us. However, I fear that in trying so hard to conceal aspects of our lives from the opposition, we also hide from one another, so losing opportunities for connection, political unity and strength.

The messages I have received about diabetes are endlessly contradictory. Apparently, if I do everything the doctors tell me, I will be 'perfectly normal'. Like so many other charities, the British Diabetic Association publishes a magazine full of encouraging, cheerful role models, while using tragic images of our lives to raise money (such as a stark, black and white photograph of a woman sticking a needle into a tiny baby: 'She has to hurt the one she loves, every day').

The women whose words you will read are not tragic figures, nor would they be better off dead. They are strong, funny, wise, friendly, independent, thoughtful, courageous, outrageous and many things besides; but they have chosen, much of the time, to talk to me of grief and loss and pain and loneliness – because no one else has asked and nobody wants to hear about these things.

One woman talks about learning 'to be more upfront about my needs, my abilities and limitations; this is a whole package'. The whole package for us, as women with illnesses, includes our sense of difference and isolation, our physical pain and weakness, as well as our emotional and political discoveries and sense of normality and ordinariness. We are special in as much as every individual is special, and we want to live in a world in which we and others are allowed to speak about the totality of our lives; a world which recognizes and accepts the good along with the bad and does not recoil in fear or seek to silence us.

In using extracts from interviews rather than producing a collection of complete interviews, I have aimed to draw out common themes in our experience. We are all very different, however, and this book is about difference as much as about commonality. Women came to me by various routes: a few are friends or friends of friends; the rest responded to publicity sent out through community groups, disability organizations, self-help groups and individual health workers. More details of the women interviewed can be found in the Biographies section, but there is no doubt that, as in many books on women's issues, those like myself – white, middle-class, youngish to middle-aged – are over-represented.

I had ambitions to reach a wider range of women than in the end I managed, but differences of race, class, age or sexuality create many barriers between us. I may have failed to get information through to some women, while others may have had good reasons for choosing not to be involved in a book of this kind. I believe, however, that the range of experience included here demonstrates how our health is affected not only by illness and disability, but also by who we are and what status the world accords to us. I hope, too, that this book succeeds in speaking to women from many different backgrounds.

Despite our differences, however, my original sense of there being many areas of common experience between women with illnesses has been borne out. One woman I interviewed rang me after reading the text and told me how many of the things said by other women she could easily have said herself. Working on this book has been a constant process of discovery of differences and similarities. I am at one and the same time overwhelmed by the differences and

## Introduction

divisions between women, excited by the connections we are able to make with one another, and amazed by the richness and range of our knowledge and experience. Together we could be very powerful.

Deciding what to include and what to exclude from the definition of chronic or long-term illness was difficult. The women I interviewed have epilepsy, arthritis, HIV (human immunodeficiency virus), sickle-cell anaemia, MS (multiple sclerosis), cancer, diabetes, ME (myalgic encephalomyelitis), lupus (systemic lupus erythmatosus or SLE), heart disease, fibromyalgia, thyroid disease, ankylosing spondylitis, spina bifida and several other less common conditions. I interviewed two women who have asthma as well as other conditions, but apart from these respiratory diseases – a major area of invisible illness – have received no mention. This was accidental rather than intentional.

I have not included injury rather than illness, nor mental as opposed to physical health problems. The latter decision was hard to justify to women who believe that anorexia, alcoholism or depression, for example, are physiologically caused, and who also feel that the separation between physical and mental illness only perpetuates the stigma attached to the latter. There are, however, already many books on women and mental health, while there are fewer on women and physical disability, and scarcely any on women with the kinds of illnesses included here. One woman in this book talks about the complex relationship between mental and physical health, an area which I do believe needs much more study. Nevertheless, the fact that her agoraphobia has been a far greater problem than the hypertension she also suffers from does make her experience different in many ways from that of other women I interviewed. There are many links to be made between the experience of women in this book and other groups of disabled or otherwise oppressed women. I hope and believe that what we have said here illuminates some aspects of all women's experience and all disabled people's experience rather than merely reflecting our own.

An important element of this book is the relationship

between the medical profession and ourselves, and my own feelings about what I have written mirror the conflicts and complexities of this relationship. Most of what women have had to say has been negative, although I certainly did not seek out people with bad experiences of health care. However, if we are dependent on doctors, as most of us in this book are in some way or other, we are frightened of offending them and also feel grateful to them. The diabetes clinic and family doctor I see at present are excellent and make me feel supported in dealing with my diabetes. Every so often, as I write bitter and condemnatory sentences about the medical profession, I feel a stab of guilt at my ingratitude towards those who help to keep me alive. However, through voluntary work on my local Community Health Council, I come up against some examples of the worst treatment the Health Service has to offer; and so often the worst is what is available to the people with least power (and least money), people who do not have the kind of choices that I do about which doctor or clinic to use.

During the last stages of writing I watched *Deadly Experiments*, a television documentary on experiments into the effects of radiation which were carried out on people in the 1960s, both in this country and in America. It left me feeling shell-shocked, angry and despairing for days afterwards. This was military research, but carried out by doctors, whose duty it is to preserve lives, not destroy them! Most of the people involved were not apparently told enough for any meaningful consent to have been given, but one group of women in Scotland were aware that the substances injected into them during pregnancy were radioactive. One of these women, Kathleen Morrison, said in an interview in the *Guardian* last year:

> We were intelligent, well-educated women who wanted the best for our children and we agreed to the tests because we never even thought that a doctor would put us at risk.[2]

*Introduction*

So often I hear doctors complaining that patients don't trust them, but I feel on the contrary that we trust them far too much for our own good. I have not reached the point of believing, as some do, that doctors and medicine are inherently harmful. I do believe, however, that genuine informed consent is virtually impossible in the context of a relationship as unequal as that between doctor and patient, or that between the medical and scientific professions and the public in general. The potential for serious abuse, including at the most extreme the taking of life, always exists. This has been said by many before me[3], but the experience of women in this book, who have dealt with doctors and the Health Service over years of their lives, provides a contemporary reminder – if one is needed – that the relationship between those of us who are sick and those we look to for our healing is one in need of drastic and fundamental change.

Finally, a few people have asked, 'Why women with chronic illness, rather than women and men?' I am not going to apologize for this, other than to say that as I am a woman and a feminist, it is women's lives in which I am interested; that from my own experience there appear to be ways in which women are affected differently from men by illness; and that women's health in general is dangerously neglected and misunderstood. More interesting, perhaps, is the way in which society's views of illness and disability are similar to its views of femininity. Both symbolize failure and weakness, as measured against the normal, male body, and, as we know to our cost, whether female or disabled or both, this means we are accorded little control over our lives and bodies. Both also symbolize the uncontrollable, mutable side of human nature, the opposite side of the coin from the active, transcendent, male experience.

While I dislike the attaching of these two opposites to female and male identity, I believe that the recognition of them both is important for all of us, men and women, disabled and non-disabled. Good health and strength allow us to turn to the outside world, to be busy, to do things and to effect change around us. Illness allows, or demands, that we be still, that we turn inwards and experience our bodies, minds and emotions more intensely. As one woman said to me, it means that we take time to breathe.

# 1

## *Feeling Different: Isolation, Invisibility and Identity*

Since 1980 I have had diabetes. Since that everything has changed for me. I can't work again. I was a nursing auxiliary and I really do miss work. I don't go out anywhere more than go to church, especially this time of the year when it gets dark. I don't know what I've done but my blood sugar's gone high at the moment. It makes me very weak and limbless and powerless over my body. Sometimes I think if you were feeling pain it would be better, but the way this thing make you feel is like you're living dead, man. You have no energy. You just can't explain to anyone how you feel. Sometimes you're out there and you're looking alright, but nobody knows what you're suffering inside.

*Joyce*

Illness is a solitary experience. Something as minor as a cold or toothache can make us feel excluded or cut off from the world, even if only temporarily. Our physical symptoms, by their very nature, are happening to our body alone and no one else can share in them. Illness reminds us that each of us is a solitary unit among other solitary units, and brings home to us the limits of human companionship and sharing. Other people may not want to be around us when we are very ill, finding us depressing or frightening. We ourselves may also need to turn inwards, away from other people:

When I'm ill I don't want anybody around. I need my energies for me and you've got to be very selfish on that point to be able to get through your day from morning till night. You need to regenerate your batteries in any way you can, then once you get through that stage you're back being positive. I don't term that as being negative, that is just my time.

*Mary*

## 'I feel different all the time': isolation and introspection

Pain and fatigue are part of the everyday experience of many of the women speaking about their lives in this book. Both these feelings tend, at least in their extreme forms, to turn us in upon ourselves. We may have periods when we are unable to relate to others or attend to their needs. Many illnesses also involve spells of disorientation and dizziness, blurred vision, or an inability to concentrate, which further affect our social interaction and make us feel different or cut off from those around us. For a time we leave the ordinary world which meanwhile carries on at its usual pace without us. This sense of dislocation and unreality may be heightened for those of us with conditions such as diabetes or epilepsy, where a temporary loss of control over our bodies is an ever-present threat. We know that healthy people, people who do not live continuously with illness, do not need constantly to keep a check on the body's functioning in the way that we do.

I want to be able to do things that other people take for granted. You have to think about everything a lot and I want to get away from that; away from 'I can't eat that because it'll set me off', 'Can I ring you nearer the time about coming to dinner because I don't know how I'll be?' and so on.

*Clare*

The ancient Romans had a god called Janus, guardian of entrances and gateways. With two faces, he looked both forwards and backwards, at the past and the future or, sat in the house doorway, at both inside and outside. I see him as our mind's eye, which must also face both ways at once, must always look inwards as well as outwards. Since our illnesses or conditions are long term, this experience of distraction, of not complete participation in the world, this solitariness to some extent or other, will become part of our everyday lives. In our dealings with people around us, we are constantly reminded of how our lives are different from theirs.

Not isolated socially, but a personal isolation of being different, like closet gay people or somebody with something to hide might feel. People assume I'm 'normal'. Then they get to know I'm different and I feel I'm sort of pulling the wool over their eyes. They'll take a step back and that's when a little bit of isolation comes over. I feel different when people say to me, 'We were up till four o'clock and then went out on a bike ride', or when people can predict their career patterns or move abroad – I think, 'Well, I can't'.

*Francesca*

I feel different all the time; like at break times, people may have a drink or a scone or something and I think, 'Well, I can't'. Sometimes I feel like I'm special because I've got this, but really I just want to feel normal, because sometimes I feel like an invisible person.

*Tracey*

When we are extremely tired or ill, we may need to be allowed to retreat. We do not have the energy to cope with the noise, the rough and tumble of other people, their joys and sorrows and need for attention. Ultimately, however, all this is the very stuff of life, and while retreat may bring peace and quiet, it also brings sadness and a sense of missing out. Audre Lorde wrote about being avoided by people when returning home after a mastectomy:

> The status of untouchable is a very unreal and lonely one, although it does keep everyone at arm's length, and protects as it insulates. But you can die of that specialness, of the cold, the isolation. It does not serve living. I began quickly to yearn for the warmth of the fray, to be as good as the old, even while the slightest touch meanwhile threatened to be unbearable.[1]

Tracey talks about feeling like an invisible person. If we are conscious that our physical and emotional experience is different from that of other people, it can leave us with a permanent sense of unease, a question mark over our very existence. It is perhaps one of life's greatest contradictions that, while each of us is an island, separate from the rest, we are not comfortable with this, constantly needing our experience confirmed and validated by other people.

## 'Something that you can't see': invisible illnesses and invisible women

Two thirds of the women in this book have an illness that is not usually obvious to others, and identify this invisibility as a major problem. Disbelief and denial of our experience are recurring themes in women's accounts of encounters with the medical profession and relationships with partners or family.

## Feeling Different

I can remember times when it would be such a relief when I got a cold, because everyone's used to people having time off work for a cold, whereas 'I'm just feeling too tired today' is a very hard thing to say. I've found, at times, I've exaggerated how I feel. I know I'm not well enough to work, but I don't know if other people are going to accept my assessment.

*Grace*

I also find that there's days when people are not very understanding, because you haven't got this stamped on your forehead.

*Bobby*

Grace talks about having time off work with a cold. A cold has visible signs, such as a runny nose or puffy eyes, so that other people do not have to rely only on our reporting of tiredness, sickness or pain. Tiredness and weakness are difficult sensations to describe, or to comprehend when they belong to someone else. Everyone feels tired at times and many women feel tired most of the time, but none of us can actually experience or assess the degree of another person's tiredness. There is considerable responsibility on the person with invisible symptoms to decide at what point they are unable to go to work, or to a party, or to pick the children up from school. We also make considerable demands on other people's trust and belief in us when we report tiredness. Similarly, pain is something that cannot be seen and the degree of pain we experience (along with our need for pain relief) is often minimized or disbelieved. Despite the fact that everyone knows pain to be very real when they experience it themselves, it is something always open to doubt or question when it is happening to someone else.

If you've got a broken leg you can lean on anybody, people will be sympathetic. But when it's something long term and particularly something that you can't see ... I feel this illness is something that you've got to cope with, because no one else can see it and nobody else can feel it.

*Patricia*

The cause of my pain syndrome can be seen on a brain scan, so there's no question of it being in my imagination.

*Eleanor*

Women frequently used the examples of a broken leg or a wheelchair as signs that were understood by others as meaning that you needed help. Marlene thinks the fact that she uses crutches makes life easier because people can see immediately that it is difficult for her to open doors or to pick up things, and so they are more likely to offer her help. Many disabled people quite rightly resent the assumptions that are made about men or women using crutches or a wheelchair. However, the other side of the coin is the frustration and loneliness of having people assume you are alright when you are not. Lesley has had a colostomy and a urostomy and so carries two bags around attached to her body. She is in more or less constant pain as a result of radiotherapy treatment for cancer, but she is young and energetic (so long as the pain is controlled) and looks like a 'normal' person:

> I parked the car at the supermarket one time and I could see this old couple talking about me, saying, 'She shouldn't park there, that's for disabled people only.' I confronted them and the woman said, 'You cannot be disabled, you're eating an ice-cream and you're walking.' And I said, 'Because I'm young and not in a wheelchair, I don't come in what you class as disabled. I have to be on morphine to make myself walk. How disabled do you want me to be?' I felt better for saying it, but afterwards I cried my eyes out.
>
> It's a terrible thing to say, but in some ways you envy the people who are sat in the wheelchair because at least

they're wearing their disability out front. You know sometimes I feel like wearing a T-shirt saying 'I have MS'. But I also think I may be frightened of telling people because then they regard me as disabled – they'll all immediately offer their seats when actually I like standing up. I suppose the people in the wheelchairs are going to get that whether they like it or not, whereas I can not tell people.

*Harriet*

People say, 'You're too good-looking to be disabled', or 'too intelligent' – mind-boggling isn't it? If I start to limp, most people will remember, other people who've forgotten will say, 'What have you done to yourself?' People assume disablement is something that you're born with, or an accident, rather than an almost invisible thing that's part and parcel of you.

*Francesca*

Many people in our society, it seems, find it hard to understand or evaluate other people's experience. We all want signs and symbols to tell us what people are and how we are supposed to relate to them. The idea of 'normality' carries with it so much that is culturally or politically defined that someone who looks normal is considered, until anything is known to the contrary, to be not simply what is visible, but also heterosexual, not disabled, not dying, not too poor, to have an occupation, a partner and a home; so many things about which there is no logical reason for us to make assumptions.

Society feels especially threatened by things that are hidden, such as homosexuality or invisible disabilities. The response that we all may meet, of people taking a step back when we tell them we have an illness, may not only be social embarrassment, but also a drawing away from contagion, from the taint of death that we bring into clean, healthy society. We may feel an unspoken accusation that we have practised deceit, that we are imposters in a normal world.

Publicity about AIDS (acquired immunity deficiency syndrome) has focused on the fact that it is invisible, that you can't tell who's got it. I saw one poster with the face of a beautiful woman concealing beneath it the face of a woman with AIDS – corruption and decay masquerading as life. Women with HIV are more feared than any of the rest of us, even in ordinary social interactions:

> My friends treated me like I was different. They don't feel they can hug or touch me.
>
> *Woman with HIV*[2]

In some circumstances, however, invisibility is considered praiseworthy rather than threatening. Not standing out from the crowd is a virtue if our visibility might place demands on others; so women or black people are praised for not making an issue of their race or gender (that is to say, of others' racism or sexism). Perhaps still more are disabled people, lesbians and gay men praised for being 'discreet' or for 'not making a fuss'. When I was first diagnosed with diabetes, I quickly learned that I was to take comfort from the idea that 'nobody need know'. I could be a 'good diabetic' by being discreet, by denying a part of myself and making few demands on those around me.

Being a woman and one with a chronic illness is only part of our identity and experience. We are black or white, heterosexual, bi-sexual or lesbian, married, single, young, old, mothers, childless, working class, middle class and so on. Yet, all other identities we might wish to claim seem to vanish, to be stripped away in the presence of illness. Once diagnosed with an illness, it is suddenly of no relevance that I am a woman (unless I wish to become pregnant). My work experience, politics or feminism are not tools that can help me but irrelevancies which will irritate my medical carers and possibly hinder me in becoming a good patient.

Information on specific illnesses rarely, if ever, addresses how it may feel to be a woman with this illness, or a black person, or someone who has another impairment, or how these identities will affect the way the Health Service treats you. In the media or in self-help literature for patients, we are presented to ourselves as generic ill people, despite the fact that the generic person in our society is, roughly speaking, a white, heterosexual man, who has little or nothing in common with many of us. Conversely, in descriptions of other aspects of life, and in information on health, we as ill people do not appear. Information on topics such as pregnancy and childbirth, miscarriage or abortion makes little or no reference to women with illnesses or impairments which might affect their feelings, medical needs or treatment.[3]

Those of us who fall into more than one marginalized group or section of society experience a particular kind of division or conflict – a total absence of any reflection of our whole self and identity. The experience of oppression and the struggle to develop positive group identities can put its own barriers in the way of recognizing the complexities of individual human existence. We may find that in our social, work or political life, we have to choose to emphasize or conceal various parts of our identity. Women talk in this book about illness but it may not be the most important aspect of our identity; rather it is one of various strands which include our gender, race, age and sexuality.

> As an older woman and a widow, I'm marginalized anyway, ill or well. I feel that the society I'm living in is all projected towards fit 25-year-olds, and the rest of us, we might as well be dead anyway. They write about someone in the paper as lonely, elderly, living in a back street, a quiet, nice woman. They could be writing about me, but that isn't me!
> 
> *Marlene*

> I see myself as disabled, but also as working class, which I think is as important. I think of equality not so much as being black or white or female or male, but still very much about the class system.
> 
> *Helen*

When I'm with my disabled friends my identity as a disabled person is at the fore and with lesbian friends it's the other way. Trying to bring one into the other is quite difficult. Disabled people are not supposed to have a sexuality, and a lot of people think that there just aren't any gay disabled people.

*Grace*

This total invisibility undermines our confidence and prevents us acquiring useful knowledge about our illness. How may we know if there is another woman out there going through the menopause with diabetes, another black woman with epilepsy, another lesbian with arthritis, another teenager with sickle-cell anaemia, or another HIV-positive mother wondering how long she has with her children? It is hard enough to forge an identity as a person with a long-term illness in a society which does not want to know about illness or impairment, but we are still more hindered in this by being rendered invisible. Black American poet, Ntozake Shange, gives a sideways glance in her play *Spell # 7* at the absence of black people in representations of illness:

> i waz young/ ... a precocious brown girl with peculiar ideas. like during the polio epidemic/ i wanted to have a celebration/ which nobody cd understand since iron lungs and not going swimming waznt nothing to celebrate. but I explained that I was celebrating the bounty of the lord/ ... it was obvious that god had protected the colored folks from polio/ nobody understood that. i did/ if god had made colored people susceptible to polio/ then we wd be on the pictures & the television with the white children. i knew only white folks cd get that particular disease/ & i celebrated.[4]

Many women talked about the need for more coverage or awareness of their particular illness in television and other media. This partly reflects the desire for other people to be better informed but, at a more fundamental level, also expresses our need, our thirst to see ourselves. If we search for, but cannot see, ourselves in the world around us, we do not know if our particular, individual existence was meant to happen, or if in fact we are simply an aberration.

# 'Climbing Everest':
## *falling short of physical perfection*

When I started with arthritis my self-image was awful. I used to wear a long coat with the collar turned up, gloves, and a trilby hat pulled down over my face. I wanted to be invisible. I used to shuffle along slowly, muttering, 'I hate you all.' I was so angry but there was nowhere for that anger to go, there was nobody saying, 'It's alright to be angry; it's going to disrupt your sense of self; all your prejudice about disability is going to turn back on you.' When I became disabled, I had to confront the way I operated a hierarchy of everybody I met. It's difficult to admit when you're a right-on, lesbian feminist with a political framework that has nothing to do with all that. But when it came down to it, there were people better than me and people that weren't as good as me, and suddenly I'd become someone worse than me.

*Grace*

We live in a society which values good health, physical fitness and 'wholeness', a society which links these with power, money and sexuality and which, fundamentally, values people for doing rather than for existing, for being active rather than passive. The normal, ideal body is that of a man, physically strong, lean and active. Women's bodies are defined as abnormal in relation to men's, and biological functions, such as menstruation or pregnancy, are seen as unhealthy, dirty and not quite human. We are not seen as effecting change in the world – the masculine, active role – but rather as passive and acted upon. We learn that others have the right to manipulate our bodies, in the interests of fashion or pornography, or in the interests of our own health.

There are parallels here with the way in which disabled people's bodies are viewed and treated. A disabled body is one which is acted upon, one which has things done to it because it doesn't function properly. We may experience surgery, tests that involve taking blood or other substances from us, or drug treatments with their side effects. Illness may also mean that we have to think more than other people around us about mundane physical aspects of existence, such as eating or excreting. Our ill bodies, like women's bodies, are therefore more animal, less sublime, and every day we are surrounded by images of thin, well, active bodies, with their implicit, negative messages about our own bodies, our limited energy levels or physical limitations.

It is hard to find a space in which to develop our own notions of achievement and fulfilment as women who have various degrees of physical limitations. So many quieter, more passive pleasures or contributions to the world around us are ignored and receive no recognition.

> I can never see myself climbing Everest, though I'd love to. I admire people who do, but I don't think I've got the courage to do something like that.
>
> *Mary*

> I wonder what I would have done with my life if I hadn't been epileptic? Yes, there are a few things that maybe I would have liked to have done – climb mountains and all that. But I'm very clumsy anyway, maybe it's as well that I don't.
>
> *Angela*

> I got it [arthritis] when I was 26, at a time when anything was possible. I had this whole list of things that maybe

one day I'd do, always this extravagant physical experience, like hang-gliding.

*Grace*

Climbing mountains, parachuting and the like are referred to over and over again by women in interviews as examples of how 'normal' people express freedom and achievement, as things which we with our illnesses cannot do, or perhaps as things we should heroically strive to do in order to demonstrate normality. Such 'extravagant physical activity' represents humankind's (or rather mankind's?) mastery over Nature and the limitations of our own bodies, symbolizing the transcendence which marks us out as different from other animals. It is a symbol that we all understand. Even when we joke about it we know that it is there, we have to go along with it or react against it.

I always fancied parachuting, but this is a girl who wanted to be a nun when she was 12! Nuns, sky-diving, it's all the same. A friend wants to take me to see this Spiritualist. You never know, it might work! Next thing you know I could be saying, 'I'm going sky-diving, a week next Tuesday.' I could probably become the first sky-diving nun.

*Harriet*

The current flock of television adverts for tampons and sanitary towels says everything to me about the aspirations and values of the society we live in, and how women and disabled people, most of all those with illnesses, can never fully live up to these. A girl skate-boarding alone on a beach – thin, young, in shorts, engaged in a typically boyish activity; a woman in tight, white shorts, climbing up ladders, jumping into a smart sports car. Using their brand of tampon or towel means that we are not really having periods at all, not really, in fact, being a woman, because to be feminine is to be weak, bleeding, suffering, not free. The white shorts deny the process of menstruation because it, like illness, is thought too unpleasant. Images of sex and violent death, on the other hand, seem to arouse less and less comment as time goes by. Hundreds of people wiped out by a robot with a laser gun is fine; a woman injecting insulin or sitting in a wheelchair upsets people. Stylized violence, involving the death of other, different people distracts us from the remembrance of our own mortality, while a disabled person or an ill person brings it closer to home.

## 'Not being a man': attitudes to disabled women

> I think it would be bloody awful if I was a man with MS. Women are supposed to be weak and helpless, so I'm just fitting into a role, being looked after by a fella. I've no complaints about being female at this point. Weak and helpless goes with women more than men, whether you like it or not, that's the way popular culture sees it. So to be a man with this disease might make you feel pretty terrible. But not being a man I wouldn't know about that.
>
> *Harriet*

How we feel about being a disabled woman or a woman with an illness depends partly on our feelings about female identity. There is no doubt that it is socially more acceptable for women than for men to be physically weak. It is also easier for women to work from home, work part time or do a mixture of paid and voluntary work, without loss of status or identity. However, if we are trying to find a more positive, more equal female identity, then becoming ill may undermine our precious independence and achievements, and throw us right back to seeing ourselves as typical weak and dependent women.

> It's hard because a large chunk of positive lesbian identity is based on being very physical, getting away from the Victorian image of the little woman who has everything done for her; but obviously there's a problem in that we are not all able to be that person – Wonder Woman striding through life, drinking and dancing all night.
>
> *Grace*

As women we also respond differently to illness than men do, usually taking our own health and illness less seriously. Society teaches us that we are less valuable than men or children, and women's responsibility for others also means that we do not often feel we can afford to be ill. So we may just carry on until unable to do so any longer. A number of women talked about men taking even minor illnesses quite seriously, and clearly expressing their need for help and sympathy. Many also thought men were encouraged in this by other people treating their illnesses more seriously than ours.

> I suppose women adapt better, because I can remember however rough I felt, especially when I had the children, you still have to get up and get going. But I've noticed with men ... they get a toothache, sore throat and they think tomorrow they're going to die. You can get a sore throat and feel absolutely knackered, but you've got a whole pile of ironing to do and a meal to get, and you just battle on through it if you possibly can.
>
> *Janet*

> My husband got a tummy bug, was very ill and couldn't keep down any fluid. So I rang the doctor. When he came he was all over my husband: 'You poor man' and far more sympathy than I'd ever had from him or any doctor.
>
> *Shirley*

> Women are expected to cope more aren't they? Like painful periods or PMT, it becomes such a part of your life that you are expected to subsume it and cope with it and not mention it too often.
>
> *Maggie*

Disabled women are also not supposed to have a sexuality. As older women know, once women are no longer seen as sexual beings, we no longer have a value for society. Men are the achievers in life and so many disabled men lose out because they can't achieve in the ways recognized as normally masculine; but many others do continue to do things for which they get recognition or status. As women, however, we are not seen as achievers, so if disabled, we may simply be seen as burdens on society, what the Nazis called 'useless eaters'. Francesca feels that since we don't fit normal ideals of womanhood, people also find us difficult as it is not obvious what we are or where we fit in:

> People can find you a bit sexually threatening in a way that they wouldn't a man, but I'm not sure why. A disabled woman is an unknown quantity, especially a single, educated, quite strong-minded one.

However Francesca has also experienced the reverse: how obviously disabled women are vulnerable to sexual abuse or violence, precisely because they are seen as even less powerful than other women:

> I got sexually harassed in a nightclub, the only time I've gone out with a walking stick, and I was absolutely gobstruck! I was standing in a crowd of people, leaning on my stick. I felt my bum being groped and I thought, 'No, it's somebody pushing past'; then it happened again, more obviously. Other women I've spoken to, particularly ones with mobility problems, have said that it's happened to them as well.

*Feeling Different*

## '*I used to get called spastic*': *growing up with an illness*

I've had epilepsy from being two years of age. My doctor told me I couldn't leave home, couldn't drink, couldn't go to nightclubs, I'd have a poor education and wouldn't be able to drive. As a child I was just massive because of the medication I was on. At school I was the only black girl, so you get noticed, and if you've a weight problem, you get noticed even more, so I used always to get 'called' because of my weight. It used to do my head in. My dad didn't understand my condition and used to always call me 'retard'. I was expected to be pregnant at 16, never leave home and do nothing for myself. So I was determined to push myself and prove I wasn't what they expected. I can't drive and I've accepted that, but I did everything else.

*Maureen*

If you have an illness from birth or early childhood, it has a very different impact on your life than if you develop it as an adult. On the positive side, you do not have a massive adjustment to go through as an adult and so are likely to be more comfortable with your illness, more clear about it being a part of yourself, rather than some alien thing foisted onto you:

I feel that being diabetic from age five, it really, genuinely is a part of me, rather than an addition, as it is for people who develop it later. Provided that I eat more or less at the same time, have got insulin in one pocket and a glucose tablet in the other, then I do what I want to do. But that's to do with a mental attitude as well. I am me and I will go where I want and do what I want.

*Helen*

On the other hand, illness may have restricted many aspects of your life when you were young. The simple fact of being different can matter more in your childhood or teens than at any other time of your life. It may have affected your sense of self-esteem as you grew up, your aspirations and ambitions, as well as what other people around you thought of you. You may have been made to feel second-rate and have grown up thinking that you could never do as well, nor ever be as good, as other 'normal' people. Alternatively, you might, like Maureen, have become determined to achieve things precisely because of the negative messages you received as you grew up, putting considerable pressure on yourself to succeed.

On a more practical level, if you missed out on education because of illness, or received a second or third-rate education – often the only kind available to disabled children – then your later education and employment opportunities will have been restricted. You may also have missed out on a lot of activities and social contact with other children. And, if you spent a lot of time in hospital, boredom and loneliness may well loom large in your memories of childhood.

> I was diagnosed as having sickle cell when I was eight. I didn't suffer many crises as a child but, from the age of eight, I lived, breathed and ate hospitals. My foot was dislocated at birth and every summer holiday I used to be in hospital on traction. That was a nightmare, because I missed a lot of schooling. There were children in with worse illnesses, but I used to think, 'Why does it have to be me? Why can't it be somebody else?'
>
> *Paris*

> When I was younger I used to be pretty slow at learning because every time I had an attack, everything I'd learned, I'd forget, and I'd have to recap. I was in and out of hospital like a yo-yo.
>
> *Maureen*

Family problems during Tracey's childhood affected her diabetes, which had also been incorrectly treated when she was first diagnosed as a baby, so it wasn't until her teens that she began to be able to manage it well:

> At school when I had hypo [hypoglycaemic] attacks I used to get called 'spastic' and stuff like that. I hated it because it was something I couldn't help and I was getting called names for it. From the age of 9 to 13, I went in and out of hospital a lot, because mum and dad kept arguing and shouting and splitting up and I got very ill. I ate too much because I was stressed and I had no one to turn to. I lived in hospital for 18 months and then, at 13, I went to a special boarding school. I hated it there, with missing my family and what have you, but it really helped me with sorting out the diabetes.

One of the difficulties for women who have had their illness all or most of their lives is that there were so many different influences operating on them as children all at the same time. As Maureen tells us, at school other children would verbally abuse her on account of her race and size rather than her epilepsy, while at home her father was calling her 'retard'. It becomes very hard, discussing all this as an adult, to distinguish which bits of your personality and upbringing are directly related to having an illness and which are not. Whether positive or negative, the illness becomes simply 'part of you'.

An additional complexity might be the recognition you may now have – as Tracey does in relation to her boarding school and Helen, below, in relation to her parents' attitudes to life – that things you disliked intensely at the time may actually have been of great benefit to your physical health.

> My parents were working class, not well off and very much into the stiff upper lip. As a child I was never allowed to say, 'It's not fair' or 'I want'. With diabetes it was: 'It's tough, but you'll have to get on with it.' The

positive side is that I'm here now. Most of my contemporaries who were diabetic are dead now because of their diabetes. My parents were strong enough to say, 'No, you can't have another piece of bread, no, you can't have anything to eat.' I was brought up not to make a fuss: don't rock the boat, don't upset anybody. It's only in the last five or six years that I've had the confidence to say what I need, that I must eat or need to stick a needle in myself.

*Helen*

Several women have conditions which they were born with but which were only diagnosed when they reached adulthood. Janet has an inherited connective tissue disorder (EDS or Ehlers-Danlos syndrome), which was not easy to trace because she was adopted:

To my parents there was no knowledge that EDS was in the family, but it can easily miss a generation. I was grateful in some respects that it did go undetected, because I was able to go to an ordinary school. I wasn't mollycoddled. I'm not saying my parents were hard on me, but I was able to do everything everybody else did as a child.

*Janet*

Adele has spina bifida and various other inherited conditions, but grew up with a violent mother who dismissed her complaints of back and leg pains. In her case, not only was she not diagnosed in childhood, but her family history became a reason for doctors not to listen to her as a young adult, so that she was in her 20s before she actually received a diagnosis (and even then her family continued to deny her disability!) So although her conditions existed when she was born, she has had to go through the same adjustments as an adult as many of us with quite different kinds of illnesses:

I started complaining of pains from the age of four. I couldn't run. If I did I always fell over. I was always being told 'Stop crying', 'Don't be such a big girl's blouse', 'Get up, you're a big girl now.' When I did get a diagnosis I had to completely reverse everything I'd ever been told. From the age of four upwards I'd always been called a liar.

## *'Pain can really bring you down': physical and emotional symptoms*

Each of us has our own individual approach to managing our illness and discovers things likely to make it worse or better. We cultivate a positive attitude and try to stay as well as possible. Some of us may even go through periods of feeling more healthy than we did before we had an illness, as we have learned how to look after ourselves. We may eat more healthily or take more rest than other people, but underneath it all we are *ill*: we have to work much harder than others to feel reasonably well and we are often in pain.

When I'm up in the night with pain, I don't have a morning, and I never know when that can be. I take morphine all the time. I get adhesion attacks which can be through something you've eaten or it can be scar tissue, but it blocks up your intestine so everything you eat comes back and your colostomy bag doesn't work. The pain is unbelievable. Some days you just have to lie on the sofa, you can't even concentrate on a book or the television. You sometimes wonder what's the point of living any more.

*Lesley*

> I have been very depressed at times, because pain can bring you very low. There were one or two occasions when I did consider, 'Well that's it, I might as well just go, there's no more point living through it.' It's usually the middle of the night and you feel very alone and isolated at that time.
>
> *Mary*

Some women, like myself with diabetes, or women with epilepsy, feel OK most of the time, but have to watch out for possible hypoglycaemic attacks or fits, which render us suddenly out of control and make us feel ill and weak. Some of us have limited energy or mobility, while others live with pain most or all of the time. Paris can sometimes avert a sickle-cell crisis before it happens, but otherwise faces days of extreme pain and a spell in hospital. ME, lupus and the various arthritis viruses can all flare up at times in response to various triggers, bringing pain and other symptoms.

Some conditions also affect our emotions, producing mood swings or depression (and, as Mary says, pain in itself makes you depressed), while others again fluctuate partly according to our stress levels and emotions. Life with illness is rarely straightforward, and is only partially within our control.

> When I get anxious my blood sugar shoots up really high and my hair gets knotty and I get eczema as well. When I feel uptight I just eat anything, just stuff it in until I feel ill. Then I think, 'Whoops!' and give myself more insulin, and so then I suffer the next day and have hypo attacks. But I'm trying to make myself relax and not worry too much.
>
> *Tracey*

> Most of the time, I know either it's my heart or the asthma, or one sets off the other. But there's days where I'm very snappy and I could cry for nothing and I don't

know what's wrong with me then. Maybe it's a low [blood sugar] after a high.

*Bobby*

Most of us find that the complex relationship between our physical and mental health is not well understood by the medical profession. It is usually something we have to learn about and cope with on our own. Sandra has high blood pressure, but has also lived with agoraphobia and depression for many years. Her experience shows how difficult it is to deal with all these different strands at once:

> It's complicated. I could do more to tackle the agoraphobia if I wasn't impaired physically by my weight. I can't do too much walking because my knees give way. Then again, I've got like this because I'm agoraphobic and so don't get my exercise, and because when I was more depressed I used to stay in bed and eat for comfort. I think my blood pressure is the least I've got to worry about, because if I only had that, I could probably live a near to normal life. Though I get days, which I think are the high blood pressure, where my head feels like something's gripping it hard like a vice, and that'll last for a few days and I can't do very much. And the beta blockers I take for blood pressure slow me down a lot; it takes me ages to get going when I first wake up in the morning. So I've a lot of things to tackle!
>
> *Sandra*

Often the most frustrating aspect of our illness is its unpredictability. Pain or tiredness may suddenly descend out of nowhere, and the quality of the fatigue that many of us experience is quite different from ordinary tiredness. It is not the sort of tiredness that will go away after a good night's sleep or if we just pull ourselves together.

> When I'm tired, it's like somebody is at the back of me and has their hands on my two shoulders, bearing me

down. That sort of tiredness, I don't know where it comes from. You're so tired you feel worthless, like it drives you out of something, you have nothing left in you.

*Joyce*

It's not a normal tiredness. Every ounce of strength that you did have goes. You end up dragging yourself around. You don't want to do anything except go to sleep.

*Sade*

Symptoms are very dependent on things like how tired you are, stress and all sorts. Some days you've got bags of energy for six or seven hours, and some days you just have no energy at all, even to go to the toilet. It's really difficult because everything has to be: 'I've got a bit of energy now, so let's go out, because in three hours from now I could be asleep.' I'm getting better but I don't think I'll ever have the same sort of energy that I had before.

*Clare*

Francesca is one of the few women who are positive about the changeable nature of illness, finding that while the 'downs' are lower than when she was well, so too the 'highs' are higher:

You get highs and lows almost to the point of slight manic depression. The highs are astonishing. You can see colours differently and get lots of ideas about what to do (sorry to sound mad!) Of course, when you're tired and ill again, it's like a drawing back, the curtain comes down again. It's better than being on an even keel.

## *'I'd like not to be so cautious':* losing freedom, confidence and control

I can't drive because the hand spasms have got worse. It's gut-wrenching that, because I was hoping to get more freedom. I now get full benefits so I can get out; it's expensive getting taxis and trains but at least I'm not forced to stay in. If I was normal, I would go walking. When I was young we used to walk for miles along beaches and I'd be crying because it hurt so much, but the sense of freedom ... I miss being able to walk.

*Adele*

Some loss of freedom, of carefreeness or spontaneity, is something mourned by all the women I spoke to. The degree of physical restriction varies enormously, from a few women who are more or less completely housebound, to others who travel, do full-time jobs and live what is called a 'normal life'. As I said at the start of this chapter, however, none of us is totally free of restriction. There is always a knowledge, more burdensome to some than others, of things we cannot or dare not do.

The thing that gets me down is that I've always got to plan two days ahead, because I've got to phone ahead for transport. It's difficult to do things spontaneously, which I'd like to do. It's sort of entered my psyche; instead of living my life in the present, I'm forever living two days ahead. I can't think, 'Oh, it's a nice day, I'll do it now.'

*Marlene*

I feel in some ways I was denied a childhood, freedom, that instant 'Let's do it!' Possibly some things never occur to me because there's that pre-thought of

'You can't do it anyway.' It's always there, never goes away.

*Helen*

The precise nature of our loss varies depending on our particular illness, our favoured areas of work or leisure, or our desires and ambitions. It doesn't matter at all to me that I cannot fly a plane or be a deep-sea diver, but it could matter enormously to someone else. Sometimes the problems are legal or financial, such as restrictions on driving or difficulties in getting insurance. Travel produces practical difficulties and anxieties for most of us:

> I think I'd be travelling a lot more. I used to travel, gallivant all over the place. But it's tiring, and if you're far away and something happens, and nobody understands or can help you with your medication, you're in big trouble. I suppose it would work out if I thought about it.
>
> *Sade*

I'd like not to be so cautious. My sister's going to Italy this year and I'd like to have gone. I'd like to just get on a plane and go. But I think as you grow older you become more cautious, don't you? In my early 20s I was a bit of a wildcat. I'd go to nightclubs all weekend, but now I find it difficult going to the pictures. I'm frightened of getting sick.

*Paris*

The element of risk is sometimes more problematic than the practical obstacles. Having an illness means being aware that our physical self is fragile. If we have already lost things as a result of our condition, we may fear further loss: of freedom, of work, of the ability to look after our children. Having one illness can also make us afraid of the possibility of another. We know that we are only human and that things can go wrong. We know that death is possible.

## Feeling Different

It was very frightening for me because it brought back the situation with my mother, finding I'd got something I'd not seen her recover from. I'd never been really ill before and I didn't have any confidence that I would wake up in the morning. I was frightened to go to sleep. It was a loss of confidence in the very essence of being. When you're younger and don't have a medical condition, you have a blithe belief that you're invincible. I probably think too much. I'm not very good at getting on with things and being brave!

*Maggie*

Anxiety can be paralysing. A key factor which will determine how much we can carry on doing things we enjoy is the degree to which we feel in control of our health. We all need to feel some degree of control, even as we come to accept the limitations on that. We all arrive at different conclusions as to how far we can influence our destiny. Marlene has found that diet makes a big difference to her arthritis and it is something she feels in control of:

I'm not supposed to eat too much chocolate, pickles, alcohol. One Christmas I did indulge in them all and I had a hell of a lot of pain. But if I go on a good diet – no pain. It really works for me. And nobody's more in control of what I eat than I am.

For many women, well or ill, our body weight and size represent control over our lives or lack of it. The desire to control our weight may be heightened if we have an illness, even though controlling it may become more complicated.

I haven't regained control over my body yet and I still have a weight problem. It's not so much wanting to be thin as being able to demonstrate control through losing weight.

*Maggie*

A lot of women with radiotherapy injuries (and I'm one of them) prefer to remain thin. It's ridiculous, we could all die tomorrow and yet we're all bothered about our weight. I think it's because it's something that we can control.

*Lesley*

We are likely to feel a greater or lesser sense of control at different times, perhaps according to what else is going on in our lives, but also depending on how well or ill we are feeling. Our confidence waxes and wanes according to how physically strong we are. When a treatment or diet, for example, is working, not only do we feel better in the present, we are also more likely to feel optimistic about the future.

I suppose I haven't got the confidence that I had before because I don't feel well enough to have that confidence in doing everything. It depends on how well you are. When I'm on the chloroquine every day I feel my illness has gone away, but it's the chloroquine that's making me feel better. Then when I go on alternate days I get a bit worse and, when I'm not on it, much worse. As I'm worse with the disease my confidence is lower.

*Shirley*

When I was on human insulin[5], I certainly wasn't in control because the hypos were worse than I'd ever experienced. In the middle of the night I would be raving and totally unaware, and my partner had to deal with that. One day I came home, lay down on the sofa and just went unconscious. In 30 odd years of diabetes that had never happened before. I felt that my independent living was being taken away, because I was reliant on my partner looking after me.

*Helen*

## Feeling Different

Some of us have conditions over which we have very little influence, and others know that diet, sleep, stress or various medications can make an enormous amount of difference. However, there is a delicate balance to be struck between finding out enough to maintain a sense of control, and avoiding setting ourselves up for failure and more anxiety. We have to accept that we cannot totally control what happens to our bodies.

I do feel in control of my life because I'm more sensible about my illness, where before I'd go out drinking and stuff like that. I do get crises now more often, but I don't do things to make me have a crisis. So I'm in control of my illness to a certain point, but if it wants to rear its ugly head, it will.

*Paris*

Sometimes I think I'm not going to live 70 or 80 years. I am not restricting my lifestyle and diet, which I should do as a diabetic. I know all the complications that I could have, but still it doesn't stop me eating biscuits. It's strange, isn't it? My husband's friend's wife died recently because of her diabetes. When I heard I was so scared – but I was still eating biscuits!

*Kabita*

I've been diagnosed HIV positive for about eight years and all that time my health has been fine. I decided a few years ago there was no point in knowing my T-cell count, but then recently I asked and they're going down. So it was like getting diagnosed all over again. It upset this wonderful illusion I had that my immune system was still working perfectly well. I've been through every healthy diet under the sun, done the lot: t'ai chi, acupuncture, Chinese herbs, vitamin pills. I'm a great believer in positive thinking. It's about getting your power back. But I've seen other people who've done all of this and they still die.

*Anna*

## 'Like a liberation?': coming to terms with illness and mortality

Once you've had cancer it never leaves you; life is never the same again. Things like standing watching the children's school play and wondering if you'll be there to see it next time. Other people would think it's silly, but you can't help thinking like that.

*Woman at a mastectomy support group*

Everybody's frightened of dying, but I'm frightened of dying young, because I haven't left my mark on this world yet. As long as life's there, you can do what you want, but once it's taken from you, you can't do anything. I think I've got respect for life. I live it to the full.

*Paris*

Being aware of the possibility of dying, or of getting older and more dependent, is frightening for everyone. If we have an illness, perhaps most of all if we have developed it as an adult, then we are very keenly aware that life may be short. For women who have been diagnosed with something such as HIV or cancer, death may seem very close from the start. Most of us, however, will find that our perspective on life and death changes. We may worry about dying before we have done the things we want to do, or we may be more concerned about the possibility of a slow deterioration and a loss of independence and control before we die.

You don't worry about dying, but about being ill and being a burden. I used to feel terribly independent; I'd live in squalor rather than go to a home, just live on tins. But I know my sons would worry so much. I suppose I'd have to go to a home, because I know the worry we had with my mother. I think everyone has fears, not dying, not even pain anymore, but just being alone.

*Rachel*

However, although the idea of death is frightening, there can be a certain liberation in looking it full in the face. It means very different things for each of us, depending partly on our illness and on our age, but many of us talked about having a sharper focus to our lives and more clarity about what we want from life.

It made me value me and my time a lot more. I can see women in jobs and relationships kowtowing to situations that are bad. I'm not saying I've used the illness as an excuse, but it makes me determined not to settle for second best, because you never know when you're going to die.

*Francesca*

HIV forced me to bring things into perspective very quickly. I had to make decisions. It's a challenge.

*Woman with HIV*[6]

The quote above comes from the survey of the needs and experiences of HIV-positive women by the London-based support organization, Positively Women, in which 60 per cent of women interviewed identified positive changes in their lives as a result of getting HIV. This did not mean that they thought it a good thing in itself, nor that they had not had bad experiences as a result of their diagnosis. It did mean, however, that getting the diagnosis had pushed them into making decisions about their lives, had made them sort out long-standing problems and change how they felt about themselves or people around them. Anna talks about this as well:

As a child I was sexually abused. It was never dealt with and was always coming out in relationships. When I was diagnosed I was able to get counselling, which was brilliant. It made me look at myself, at everything. It made me stop drinking or taking any hard drugs. It made me look at my family life and appreciate it so much more, because it's so delicate, it could just go tomorrow.

ME is less obviously life-threatening than HIV, but for many women involves a long initial period of being extremely ill, which is also likely to change how they think about their lives:

In a way, getting ME was like a liberation because it enabled me to come out as ill, rather than pretend to be a well person and struggle to keep up with what other people did – work full time, have friendships and go out – which I barely managed. Once I got ME I was able to say, 'Right, this is why.' I have a justifiable reason for me. It was almost a relief. I'm more powerful, I think, more my real self, not having to struggle to be something which was a lie.

*Jessie*

It's given me time to think, time for myself, which has been important. I was quite young when I became ill, so you grow up. I feel a lot calmer. I've learned to put myself first, whereas before I'd take on things that I didn't want to do but felt I should do. I see things in a different light because I've had to do things so slowly and been able to see nothing but the walls of my bedroom. I used to live life so quickly, with no time to stop and take breath and evaluate.

*Clare*

For some women, time to reflect is perhaps the most important gain from a period of illness: time to think about ourselves and what we are doing, perhaps to think about the reasons why we are ill, and what this may tell us about who we are and who we want to be.

## Feeling Different

> I had been driving myself in a direction that didn't really suit me. I wanted to be part of a sort of surrogate family, a culture, and one of the ways that I could do that was being out there partying, drinking, dancing, all of that. When I got arthritis it was like an enforced withdrawal. It gave me breathing space at a time when I was quite unhappy but had a facade of having a good life. I had vague ideas that I ought to be more successful, more popular and more happy than I was, but I wasn't actively doing anything about it.
>
> *Grace*

Giving up trying to live up to other people's standards, or even to standards which we imposed on ourselves, is one of the main areas in which some of us have changed. Physical appearance and the appearance of our houses are key areas in which women are judged and encouraged to compete. Although some of us have found it very depressing not to be able to keep our houses as clean as we could when we were healthier, others of us have begun to change our perceptions of how important housework is, or whether we are doing it for ourselves or for others.

> My attitude is that if by any chance the cleaning hasn't been done and they're going to criticize, I'll just turn round and say, 'Well you get a duster and do it yourself. You haven't come to see the dust, you've come to see me.' If they can't take me as they find me, then sorry, they're not worth knowing.
>
> *Janet*

Grace has also found life easier since thinking about what she wants for herself, rather than trying to live up to other people's ideas of achievement:

> I'm much more honest with myself. Do the fuck I want to go hang-gliding! I would rather fly a kite and I can fly a kite. My nan would say something about cutting your coat

according to your cloth, which is about acceptance. I think before I got arthritis there wasn't a lot of that around.

We tend to take our health for granted until we experience serious illness, and it comes as a shock to find that we can't necessarily do everything we thought we could. Some of us have taken getting an illness, very simply, as a sign that we were doing too much. An 'official' illness or condition gives us permission to do less or to do different things. It may also make us see more clearly what things about our lives, and what people in them are good or bad for us. Besides feeling more like her real self, Jessie also found that her partner's complete inability to support her when she was at her most ill was the spur to make her leave an unhappy relationship. Similarly, Eleanor's stroke in her mid-20s was the most important turning point in her life:

> I was sustained by the fact that I'd left my ex-partner. I used to think that no matter how appalling things were, I didn't want to go back, because it was so fantastic that I'd been able to leave. I realized that I should have left a long time previously.
>
> *Jessie*

> It was the best thing that ever happened to me. My life up till then had been bloody awful. All through my childhood I had suffered a form of abuse based on my parents religion. I woke up one morning, lying there in hospital, paralysed, and I suddenly knew that if I was going to live like this, life was going to have to be worth living, and that the only way I could make it worth living was to get the family off my back. So I went straight from hospital to my own flat and life has been a great deal better ever since. At least now I can look people in the eye and if they don't like me, it's me they don't like, not this character that's been stuck onto me by somebody else.
>
> *Eleanor*

This road to acceptance may be a long and hard one, however, and we may experience great anger or despair.

> I had to go through a phase of great pain and negativity: not wanting to be alive, not wanting anyone else to be alive either, and certainly not wanting anyone to be alive and fit and running around having a good time!
> *Grace*

Adele spent years fighting to get a diagnosis of her condition, in the hope of treatment or a cure, only to find that there was none:

> I'll never forget, I was in the park. It was a beautiful day, all the birds whistling and twilliping away, and I thought, 'That's it, I'm disabled.' It was the most gut-wrenching moment, as if someone had turned the volume of life down. I was one step removed from life, as if I was watching somebody else. It took six years for it to really sink in, and even now I'm fighting it.
> *Adele*

Adele's various conditions (including spina bifida and arthritis) have deteriorated over the years, but the fact that she has managed to get appropriate benefits and care cover has changed her life greatly for the better. The degree of struggle necessary to get these needs met has also made her less hard on herself:

> The more relaxed I am the less pain I'm in. It's just listening to what my body says it wants. I used to be so tired, felt I was a failure, because I had to live up to all these standards. I spent two years trying to get the specialists and the money sorted out, trying to get somebody to come and check me every morning, and then everything fell into place. Now I don't have to live up to anybody's ideal.
> *Adele*

We each use different language to describe these changes and struggles. We might call it personal growth, spiritual development, or just learning to love yourself. When the going is tough, some of us gain strength and comfort through therapy, others through politics or religious faith.

> There are two ways of looking at it. You can feel very sorry for yourself or you can make the best of it. There's always somebody worse off, and I see it when I'm out and about. Some people say, 'If you're a Christian, do you not blame God for the position you're in?' And yes, I did once, if I'm honest, but I got over that. Now I'm just grateful for the encouragement, support and friendship that I've had from the church I go to.
>
> *Janet*

> I don't like to say I'm fed up. I think that's a strong word for a Christian, but this illness makes you feel helpless and hopeless. It scares you to death. A woman I know had two legs amputated because of this wicked thing and it makes you think, my God, what next, who next? But I just live day by day as it comes. I don't look overboard for things, I just wait to see what the Lord will do. I trust in him and believe that whatever he will do, that will be right.
>
> *Joyce*

## 'A normal, everyday thing': part of our identity

Somebody asked me, 'If they find a cure for sickle cell, would you be one of the first in the queue?' I said no, because I've lived with this illness for so long, I don't think I'd want to be cured. I was born with it, it's part of me. I'd like to have good health, but I wouldn't want to be anybody else other than me. So it's a normal, everyday thing to me, like the way I walk. People say, 'Doesn't she walk funny?' – but I don't see myself walking funny. I don't see myself as having a handicap or a disability. I just see myself as being normal.

*Paris*

Ultimately we all have to find our own kind of peace with ourselves and our illness. Those who have had a particularly hard time, who are no longer able to do the things that meant most to them, or who feel that their present ill health could have been avoided through better diagnosis or treatment, may feel more bitter or a greater sense of loss than others. Many of us said that our initial resentment or anger wore off with the realization that many people had more serious conditions, or were worse off in other ways. This may seem rather cold comfort, but is perhaps simply another way of saying that having an illness makes us much more keenly aware of all of life's possibilities, all its joys and griefs. We mourn the things we have lost but, taking nothing for granted, appreciate what we do have perhaps more than those who are well and have never been ill. And in the end, what choice do we have?

I've come to terms with it because I don't think I have any alternative. It's not been easy, but I was always a strong-willed person. It's going to get me one day, but I'm going down fighting. I've had a very good innings. I had my first lump removed in 1968, a mastectomy 16 years ago, and a lung taken away 7 years ago. I don't feel ill. I play golf, play bridge, do my housework, sewing or whatever. I'm one of the lucky ones. So many people don't get this opportunity.

*Woman at a cancer support group*

It's tough, just the luck of the draw. There are much worse things.

*Angela*

I've not felt lonely because I've got a lot of inner resources. I think you lose some self-esteem. The main thing is the frustration of not being able to do things. I'd like to be gardening and travelling. Two unfulfilled ambitions: to go hill-walking in Nepal and to visit a friend in Australia. I don't think I'll do either now. I'm getting to that age when friends are dying, so it makes you glad that each day is a bonus. You make the most of what you've got.

*Rachel*

On the whole, the longer we live with our illness, the more inseparable it becomes from the rest of our lives and our personalities. As we grow older, we look back at the good and bad breaks we have had and good and bad choices we have made. There are so many 'What if?'s to which we will never know the answers. We have time to reflect on the influence of illness. For some of us, it has changed our lives out of all recognition, for good or bad or both; for others, it is simply one major influence among several.

I love to watch the sunset. I can't see it from my flat and I'd love to be able to stroll out for a look, but then I think young, strong women don't like walking about because they don't feel safe. My life could have been worse, could have been better. Sometimes you look in the mirror and think 'Who's that old lady there?' and it's me! So a lot of my life is intertwined with getting older. I might be happier now with arthritis than I would be without it, who knows? I suppose it has given me more time to think, but I was always the sort of person to think. I try to be positive, and no matter what happens, I try to make a life for myself.

*Marlene*

## Feeling Different

I have great trouble remembering how I was when I was fit. Things have not gone according to plan because of the rate at which I'm deteriorating. It would be nice to have my life now without it, to have it taken away, but stay as I am, as it's made me.

*Eleanor*

In the end, we are all simply women, as ordinary or extraordinary as any of you reading this book. We have talked about being invisible, being different, being seen by other people as second-rate, or depressing, or as symbols of death or decay. But we are not symbols. We are just ourselves, perhaps with a little more to think about than people who are well. We wake in the morning, feel better on some days than others, are happy when the sun is shining, sorry when the day is wet and cold. We eat, sleep, work, love our children and partners, talk to our animals and plants, go to church, paint pictures, clean the house. We could do without the pain and tiredness, the indigestion from the drugs, the mood swings, the stiffness or poor vision. We know, as who should know better, the value of good health; but we know our own value too.

I just live my life, just get on with it. That's how I think about both being a woman and being disabled. You just have to get on with it. I stand up for myself and if somebody's going to try to put me down I'll say, 'Look here, I'm an individual and I'm a person just the same as anyone else.' I don't know what else you can do.

*Mary*

I love me. I am very willing to help other people and I treat everybody with respect. I reckon that makes me a nice person. I think I'm quite worthwhile, which after an upbringing like mine says an awful lot. It's taken me a lot to realize that I'm not everybody's servant. I'm an independent person with rights and I can demand those rights. God help the rest of the world because I'm out now!

*Adele*

## 2

# *Feeling Useful: Work, Roles and Contributing to Society*

**W**e are measured by our ability to work, our ability to perform and to do things that contribute. If you're disabled, you don't do those things and you don't have a right to all sorts of things because of that. I'm a nobody because I don't contribute to society.

*Clare*

I find it difficult to say no if somebody asks me to do something. You want to help. You want to feel useful and there's times when you don't feel useful. It can be quite despairing at times to think that you're never going to work again.

*Mary*

We may see ourselves as ordinary people and ordinary women, but one of the main definitions of normality in our culture is work. In spite of the fact that there are many people who can't get work, not working is still seen as something needing explanation. So often the first question anyone asks of a new acquaintance is: 'So, what do you do?' It is one of the ways in which we place people. Workers may often be exploited, but they have a recognized place in the world. Besides an identity and status, work also provides social contact and an income. If we are not able to work because of our illness then we may lose all of these.

## Feeling Useful

Fewer than a quarter of the women I interviewed were working full time when I spoke to them or are doing so now. The majority do some amount of part-time, freelance or voluntary work. Two of the three women who are currently at home looking after children would like to have outside work but are not well enough.

During their lives the women have worked in many different fields: nursing, libraries, public relations, the civil service, teaching, shops and supermarkets, launderettes, dentistry, the hotel industry, clerical work and the charitable and voluntary sector. We have also been involved in disability campaigning, community work, local politics and trade unions. Our current work, paid and unpaid, includes: housework, the care of our own children or grandchildren, paid child minding, studying, writing, university teaching, social and community work, being a Justice of the Peace and advice or campaigning work with women and disabled people. Several of us also spend time on music, drama, art, craft, walking, looking after pets and so on.

Most of us at some point have had to give up work or reduce the amount we do as a result of a deterioration in our health. Illness may also have caused us to change the sort of work we do. Those of us who can afford some choice may now be finding voluntary or campaigning work more fulfilling than we did our previous work. No matter what our level of income and activity, almost all of us would like to be more active than we are and (other than those who have already reached retirement age) most of us would like to be working more than we are. We need the money and we miss the daily contact with people, the confidence and sense of being involved in the world which work can provide.

> I would love to be able to work. I worked in a school for handicapped children and I used to do newspaper rounds and work in a shop. I loved shop work because you get to meet so many people. I miss that.
>
> *Adele*

I think I've diminished. I've got less to say for myself. I've got very little opinion of myself and I blame that partly on the illness, because it stops you going out to work. As the kids have got older, I might have gone back to work, something extremely demanding like serving in a shop. But now I couldn't do that.

*Harriet*

It worries me a bit that I might never be able to work full time again. I like having a project in hand and I like earning and spending money. It's a bit of bummer really. I can't plan any sort of career structure, as I wanted to do after I graduated as a mature student.

*Francesca*

Because I don't have a job I don't interact with people in the ways that everyone else does, so your self-confidence does take a bit of a battering.

*Clare*

A common myth in our society is that people become ill or take sick leave because they are lazy or can't cope with the pressures of the rat race. This picture bears no relation whatsoever to the lives of women in this book, who are all very busy within the constraints of what their bodies and energy levels allow. For most of us, or for our families, problems are often caused by our trying to do more than we can manage, rather than less.

## 'Can you dress yourself?': prejudice in employment

While we may have different feelings or ambitions about our work, it is an ordinary and basic human desire to wish to do something with our time, to be useful, to interact with other people and not to be bored. However, the society we are living in puts extreme pressure on people to fill up all of their time, to achieve certain goals and to earn as much money as possible.

For many years now, economic stresses and reductions in staff levels have been putting great strain on those still in employment. There is decreasing choice about work patterns and decreasing tolerance of sick leave.[1] Talk of 'flexibility' often thinly conceals cost-cutting, diminished commitment from employers and reduced security for employees. Current working practices are only fit for those who are strong and well and, despite some increased awareness of equal opportunities issues, today's climate is profoundly hostile to the employment of people who may in any way be seen as 'not fit' or a 'problem'. Maureen and Eleanor have both experienced the prejudice employers often display towards disabled people:

> Job-wise I've had no luck. I worked in a launderette on Saturdays. I left that because of getting my disability benefits: they'd say I'm fit to work and so not give them to me. I did a Diploma in Caring and worked in an old people's home, but once they found out I took fits they didn't keep me on. What annoyed me was that they're alright to employ you when you work for nowt (on placement), but when you want to be on the payroll it's another story. I've tried my hardest. One thing people can't put me down for is trying, because I've always been a tryer. It's not that there aren't jobs, it's just that people

won't accept you if they can take someone without a medical condition.

*Maureen*

I used to waver between admitting that I was disabled on the application form and not putting it on – but then I had to be prepared for the reaction when I walked into the interview room. Their faces would change and they'd start tacking a 'dear' onto the end of every sentence. I was often asked, 'Can you dress yourself?' – obviously not one of the routine interview questions. And that was with a CV saying that I live on my own, that I'd been working for so many years doing this job. And I knew my references were good.

*Eleanor*

Studying is one way to occupy ourselves and gain qualifications which may help us to find work more easily. But we cannot study forever. Maureen feels that she has studied enough now. Eleanor, too, feels that all her qualifications should have led to some work, but she has been let down by the deterioration in her condition and the shortage of part-time university teaching:

I could go back to college and do A levels, but I've got all these certificates already and there's people getting work with not even half that. For the type of work I want to do, I'd be over-qualified if I got A levels. I want to work with disabled children because I think people like me, who have a medical condition, are more responsible and can understand what it's like better than people who haven't.

*Maureen*

I went and did a degree when I was 35 and then an MA and a teaching certificate. Now I'd like to work and earn some money. I don't want to sit at home being a very well-educated vegetable, but at the rate that I'm deteriorating I don't know how long I could hold a job down because I get so exhausted.

*Eleanor*

Angela found it relatively easy training and working as a dental surgeon, but her epilepsy did tell against her in getting a job at first:

> I had decided on my career before I had my first full-blown attack. It never dawned on me that it wasn't the right thing to do. I was accepted at hospital and had one attack in Lyons Corner House and the hospital suspended me for six months. They let me finish, but they didn't offer me a job, and if you don't get a job at your own hospital, you don't get a job in London. I went to Belfast and was on 24-hour duty for six months and I coped, didn't have any attacks. Only once in all the years I was working did I have an attack at work. The nurse knew about me so she knew to get the patient out of the chair and that was it.

Angela and Mary both feel that gender was probably a bigger problem in their work life than their illness:

> I think it's mainly because I'm a woman that I haven't been able to do the work that I wanted. I applied to train to do maxillo-facial work and they wouldn't have me, said they didn't have facilities for women. I said I could share the nurses' facilities but they still said no. I didn't want to be paid even, I just wanted experience. All the time I was studying I'd never seen a broken jaw; then I get to Northern Ireland and I'm fixing them right, left and centre. It's a dentist's not a doctor's job and I had it down to a fine art – but they wouldn't take me and they didn't know about the epilepsy, as far as I know.
>
> *Angela*

In the past I have mostly worked in service industries, and being a woman in that environment, it's much easier for people to step on you. Now I am a Justice of the Peace and as a woman in court you have to be very assertive. Some of my colleagues are very helpful and sometimes you're totally ignored.

*Mary*

But prejudice is not the only problem. On a more practical level, the disabled people's movement has often focused on the lack of physical access to buildings as a key issue in relation to employment. Several of us are unable to climb stairs or can only do so with difficulty, so the question of access is obviously important at work or where we study:

> They just don't allow for people with disabilities at all, you're expected to just get on with it. Parking's a problem, steps, just everything. At court they ignore the fact that you have a disability.
>
> *Mary*

I am lucky in that I've worked mainly in organizations run by disabled people, where there's a much higher understanding of both the physical and organizational barriers to work. When I went and did a course at a university recently, I found myself in a totally inaccessible environment in every possible way, so that was a bit of a shock to the system.

*Grace*

*Feeling Useful*

## 'Colleagues think I'm lazy': pressures on other people

If you do manage to get work or hold down a job, your problems are not over. Several women have had to confront either disbelief or unsupportive and cruel behaviour from work colleagues. It is especially distressing if we work in an area where we expect to get more support. Sade was diagnosed with lupus after many years of unexplained symptoms and medical tests. Returning to her nursing work after the near-fatal lupus flare which had finally led to the diagnosis, she was faced with total denial of her illness by her workmates:

> They thought I was just being lazy and slow: 'Everyone's tired', that's what I was told when I tried to explain. Eventually it got so bad I spoke to one of the managers and he had a word with them, but they didn't like that. They wouldn't speak to me, sent me to Coventry for two weeks. They're better now, since I got them some leaflets about lupus. I think they were horrified to read them, but now they deny that they said those things to me, that they were so horrible to me.

Shirley, who also has lupus, used to be a health visitor, and was surprised at the inflexibility of the Health Service as an employer – she had to retire, rather than working part time as she would have preferred:

> I felt that they could be more sympathetic to someone who's got a chronic illness, and not be in such indecent haste to get rid of them. If they didn't put such a lot of work onto you, you could maybe manage, but they expect such superhuman effort from you. I wouldn't think the Health Service is the place to work with a

chronic illness. I know they're under so much pressure and financial stress, but it's not very fair really.

She, too, was surprised and hurt at the attitudes of her colleagues:

> After I left I went back once to a party for someone else who was leaving. It was quite unpleasant. People were very strange, as if they thought that if I was well enough to come to the party, I was well enough to have stayed on at work (although it had cost me an enormous effort to get there). I decided not to go back again.

The inability of colleagues to accept our illness may well stem from resentment about their own unmet needs. Sade's colleagues said, 'Everyone's tired', which, among overstretched and under-paid nurses, must be true. If we have to take on less work, or do some things more slowly, it may also mean others doing more and this will cause panic if people already feel overloaded. Similarly, there is an unspoken resentment in many offices towards women (or occasionally men) who leave on the dot of 3.00 p.m. to look after children. Once you cross the line from health to illness, once you have succeeded in getting a label, then you have some permission not to do things, or not to be at work, while others who still count as 'well' have to keep going. The more tired or pressured, the more likely other people are to find reasons to resent or minimize your illness. While larger employers may be putting increasing pressure on people with health problems these days, many smaller organizations have always been understaffed and overworked, and it is hard not to feel guilty if you are less well than others:

> My memory went and when I came back to work I was misfiling things and forgetting things. This pissed people off, although they were trying to be sympathetic and supportive. No one realized at that time that it was actually a symptom of my illness. Things would get pretty

tense. I still get very tired and I have learned to accept that if I feel ill or tired I have to go home early. But that's really hard to do in a small organization, where if one person isn't working then it has an effect on everybody else.

*Jasmin*

If you live with a long-term illness it's a daily, well, a constant process of assessment as to whether or not you are well enough to do things, and you don't always know if other people are going to accept your assessment. Obviously I'm the one that knows best, but in small organizations there is a lot of pressure from other people. Working in theatre there's an expectation that, if you're committed to it, you'll give all the hours possible. When the problem is fatigue rather than more obviously not being able to do something, it is quite difficult to negotiate.

*Grace*

There is a contradiction in that I work in the voluntary sector in a supposedly caring environment (and really over the top on equal opportunities!), but in practice, it's a bloody nuisance for people. In the stressed kind of places that we're in at the moment, I know that I've irritated people sometimes by calling for a break or calling a meeting to an end (because I need to eat), and they're not always quick enough to hide it. I'm strong enough to come out and say it, whereas the quieter or more mousy person wouldn't.

*Helen*

Many people who may be aware of issues such as physical access still don't see invisible conditions, such as diabetes or epilepsy, as causing genuine disability.

I know that I got some jobs because I am registered disabled and employers have to fill a quota, and it was 'Oh well, diabetics are alright as long as they have their insulin and eat.' But on the other hand, I think that when there's a problem with diabetes, it's a big problem – like somebody collapsing on the floor or doing something dangerous with machinery.

So many of us who look 'normal' may initially appear to be less trouble for employers than other disabled people who need equipment or building adaptations, or who might frighten the customers! When it turns out, however, that we do have different needs from other workers who are not ill, colleagues and employers may well feel cheated and make us feel very guilty. Grace has lived and worked with rheumatoid arthritis for 10 years and feels she is gradually learning to be less apologetic about her needs:

> I'm going to be much more upfront about what my needs are, and my abilities and my limitations. This is a whole package. When I haven't done that in the past, I've felt very guilty introducing it at a later stage, saying that I need a rest or that the room isn't warm enough for me to work in. I'm able to do that now, partly because I have more confidence in what I *can* do than I ever did before. I used to concentrate on what I *couldn't* do.

If some of us have problems working in relatively liberal sectors, such as charities or theatre, how do we fare if we work in more traditional, less well-paid and less high-status areas? Tracey, who like Helen has had diabetes from an early age, had problems when she worked on a supermarket checkout.

> Some customers are alright, but I've had a couple complaining when I'm on the checkout and I've had a hypo. I can understand their point of view, they just want to get out, but I'm just trying to sort myself out so I can carry on serving and not pass out in front of them.

Tracey eventually left this part-time job after a few years, as she felt that her employers didn't want her there. They were obstructive about her taking breaks at particular times to eat and do injections, and refused to allow her to keep a sugary drink or chocolate bar with her on the checkout (so that she could deal with a hypoglycaemic attack quickly). They eventually reorganized shift times to allow for even fewer breaks, and announced a crack down on employees taking too much sick leave. The long hours on the checkout and the stress of fighting them had a disastrous effect on her diabetes.

Paris is very afraid of losing her job as a result of having frequent periods of sick leave:

> Every time I get sick, I think to myself, 'Am I going to lose my job this time?' And that's what I fear more than anything. I like my little place, I like my freedom, I like having a car – to lose all that would be awful. Work [as a residential social worker] is important to me. I feel I have a lot to offer children. To take my work away would be like chopping off my arm. It gives me something to do in life.

It is not just that she loves her job, however, she also feels that her illness gives her something positive to contribute to her work:

> I'm seen as being one of the members of staff who can cope with children who come into our care and have disability problems, as someone who can cope with anything they throw at me. That's the way I see myself as well. The kids accept that now and again I get ill and have to stay in hospital. If they were living at home with a parent who got sick it would be no different, so it's more like real life than putting four healthy members of staff in there. So I think I play a part where I work. I'm glad to play that part and my colleagues know that I work to my full potential when I'm there.
>
> *Paris*

## '*A little bit of strength*': the energy factor

Some women are still working, capable of doing a full-time job, but worried about the long-term effect of working so hard:

> Since I knew about my T-cell count going down I've started wondering if I should work full time. Maybe I should stop work, get a dog and stay at home and bake, and be there for my son when he comes home from school.
>
> *Anna*

Anna has been involved in support work with other HIV-positive women who have similar worries:

> Women are poor, that's the other thing. Most women I've seen haven't got work, haven't got an income. They're on social security and they need money for lots of reasons, to pay the bills, but also to get good food. Getting disability benefits is very difficult because you have to have a certain T-cell count and your doctors have to cooperate. And with HIV some people, who used to be able to do that extra cleaning job to pay the bills, don't feel like doing it anymore because they're worried that it might affect their health.

Women who know they are HIV positive have perhaps a particularly complicated task in working out what changes to make to their lives. While there is much to fear for the future, many women, like Anna, do not actually feel ill for many years. So the question is whether or not the amount of work they do will have any impact on the progress of the disease and how long they live. In some ways, the women I

## Feeling Useful

spoke to with ME are in almost the opposite situation: they have started by being extremely ill, but expect gradually to get better and to be able to do more than they do now, even if not as much as they used to do before becoming ill.

So, for many of us, the greatest problem in relation to work is our limited physical energy. Easier physical access and comfortable working conditions could obviously alleviate problems, but the number of hours worked is probably a more important factor for most of us. Some of us feel that we could have carried on working if employment was more flexible, for instance, if we had been able to work part time from the early stages of becoming ill. We have talked a little in the previous chapter about the kind of fatigue and tiredness many of us experience. This lack of energy affects all our activities, such as hobbies, voluntary work or housework, as well as paid employment. We have to learn to prioritize tasks and ration our energy carefully.

> I'd say that I have about 60 per cent of the energy that I used to have. If I'm trying to decorate the house, three hours' work would be the most I could do in a day.
>
> *Grace*

> I want to go and wash some clothes or sweep down the stairs, but you just look at it and walk off because you have no energy for it. I used to get up in the morning and by the time it was light I would have washing on the line – but not now.
>
> *Joyce*

> Some days I can move the earth but others I can't peg a line of washing. I'm frustrated that I can't do the things in the house that I've always done. Just everyday life is at a slower pace than I want it to be.
>
> *Patricia*

Often it is not just our actual limitations which drive us demented, but the changes and unpredictability in how our bodies behave. It is this uncertainty more than anything which makes some of us feel not in control and unable to take on many tasks:

> You can't plan a day ahead. You can't plan in the morning what you're going to do in the afternoon. I hate that, but now it's just the only way to live. It's no good saying my body's not in control because I'd just be lying. I feel I'm just a speck in the order of things because I can't be relied on to do anything.
>
> *Harriet*

We all get frustrated by not being able to do more. As Mary says, 'You want to feel useful.' Our insistence on undertaking more at times than our physical strength may allow can be infuriating for people around us, who simply can't understand why we are not more realistic. But it is so boring, so tiresome being able to do less than we want to, less than we are used to, that we often resist this knowledge.

> On good days I tend to feel full of false hopes which are easily shattered soon afterwards.
>
> *Francesca*

> I should rest more, but if I feel a little bit of strength I'm off to look for somebody, just for company's sake or to get out of the house.
>
> *Joyce*

When we are ill it is almost impossible to imagine being well again, and when we feel well we almost forget how it feels to be ill.[2] This is perhaps why every bad day or spell of illness is like a brush with death: we cross a line, feel life and energy ebb away. Then as strength returns, as we feel a surge of well-being, we can believe ourselves cured and take on tasks or activities accordingly.

And I'll take three Co-dydramol and for a couple of hours, for that brief space of time, I am pain-free. I promptly go mad and do all the jobs I couldn't do before and then I'm in pain again.

I make things worse by doing things that I know are not really very sensible. I think, 'Oh, I'll paint that door frame, it'll take me about 10 minutes.' I get the brush out and after a bit I can't hold my arms up any more. So I stand on a chair and do a bit more and I'm in tears trying to finish it, because I know that you can't leave a frame half-painted and that when my husband comes in he's going to have to do something straight from work that I shouldn't have started in the first place. But I always think, 'It's going to be different today, I'll be able to do that.'

*Patricia*

Because I was at home, I felt I had to do things like laundry or cleaning, which was ridiculous because I didn't have the energy. If I did one load of laundry, I'd be out completely for two whole days. I think we're all brought up with quite strong ideas of how everyone should be really well.

*Jasmin*

Our desire still to be active, still to have a role and purpose in life, partly reflects dominant social values, the fact that society does not value those who do not act and are not busy. If we have developed our illness as an adult or have a condition that is deteriorating, and if we have been used to being very active, our self-image and identity may be very much tied up with this, making it hard for us to adjust. We may make necessary changes but still often find ourselves doing too much:

My life now revolves around a lot of voluntary work. I need to be able to choose. I think everyone has to find a balance. I just couldn't do something eight hours a day, every day. Even with voluntary work I still find at times that you push yourself too hard, and you know when you do: 'Right, I'm going to be ill for the next couple of days.'

*Mary*

Sometimes I think that on good days I do more now (for the support group) than when I was working, and I wonder why I do it. But I was like that with my trade union work before I was ill, so that's just what I'm like. I've felt I had to do it because I've come across so many women who don't have the education or skills to fight back.

*Lesley*

## 'Living like a duchess': positive changes

Quite a few women I spoke to have changed their work patterns, or at least thought about doing so, as a result of becoming ill. For some this has not been entirely negative. The realization that we can no longer manage a full-time paid job, or at least not do so without further damage to our health, may stimulate or force us to find greater fulfilment elsewhere and to try new things. Marlene worked for many years and is very conscious of the greater flexibility and choice she now has in her life:

If I hadn't got arthritis, I would have continued teaching and probably had a nervous breakdown by now. In an extraordinary way my life is much better, because I've got the leisure. I say to people sometimes that I'm living like a duchess, because every week I pick out what I want to go to, the things that are free, and I book up the transport and I go. Tomorrow I'm going to the Flower Show. I go to a couple of art groups and a lot of craft exhibitions, and I'm on two or three committees. So I'm very busy really.

Perhaps it is easier for Marlene and other older women to value their leisure, having already worked for many years:

There's so many people out of work, even young, fit people. I feel sorry for them, because when I was young I could get a job anywhere, and if I didn't like it I'd just leave and get another job. In my whole long life I've seen so many changes, and living in London now is like being on another planet. This week I've just started a computer literacy course.

Angela has been doing voluntary work with a disabled people's organization since she retired. She has found it not only interesting, but also that it has changed her perspective on disability:

Through a friend who is a social worker I got involved with the local Association of Disabled People and worked on their information. When they decided to set up an advocacy consortium I became part of the steering committee. I've been chair now for seven years. I never thought of myself as disabled when I was younger, it never dawned on me. Until someone who is epileptic came to give a talk, I never knew if people counted it as a disability.

Several of us also feel that more possibilities and a greater flexibility exist for women with an illness than for men, since our identity is not so wholly linked to our job. It is possible for us to work part time or from home, to do a mixture of paid and voluntary work, or just voluntary work, without feeling we have lost all our previous status. Most women are also used to managing several different identities or roles at the same time; they may be mother, office worker and volunteer all at once. Those who particularly enjoy their profession, or earning money, or perhaps those who, due to their age or class background, grew up assuming that women had important jobs, may find their identity more linked to their work and so find it harder to adjust. Most women, however, have other roles which are as important their jobs.

> My husband wasn't able to cope with his illness the way I've coped with mine. He was his job, like a lot of men are. Once their job is finished they can't see themselves in some other role, whereas I think I could find some sort of a role whatever comes up.
>
> *Marlene*

> I've been quite lucky that I've been at home and able to do what I want within my limitations. It would be hard to be a man with AS [ankylosing spondylitis], trying to go out to work with it.
>
> *Mary*

## 'Not so terribly important': a lack of support for women

Not all of us, however, have experience and skills that are transferable to part-time or home-based work. Some of us, particularly those with responsibility for others, may find that limiting what we do involves cutting out the things we want to do for ourselves, since housework or paid work takes up all our energy.

> In the morning when I get up my mind's got all the things in it that I want to do and at the end of the day

they're all still there because I've only managed to achieve one or two. There's things I want to do outside the house, like doing something with the elderly in the community, that I don't do because it's taking energy that I need for the kids and the house.

*Patricia*

Some choices may also not be open to us, or may be made more difficult, because of the way the benefits system works:

> It keeps me sane, this voluntary work, but on saying that I was pulled for doing it. I had to get a note from the doctor to say it was therapeutic, otherwise I could lose all my benefits. Silly, isn't it? Sometimes I can't be here [at the community centre] for two or three weeks, and that's fine, but if you're in a job you can't do that. And it stops you vegetating, keeps your mind going. Most of these places couldn't run without volunteers and it's mainly disabled or elderly volunteers who do the work.
>
> *Bobby*

Maureen gave up her Saturday job in a launderette because doing this for one day a week would mean she qualified as fit for work and so would not get benefits. However, the fact she might be fit enough to work doesn't stop employers discriminating against her because of her epilepsy. Living on basic income support, without disability benefits, is pretty unhealthy for someone who is well, and how much more so for someone who is already ill? As Bobby mentions, there is provision for doing 'therapeutic' voluntary work or a small amount of work for 'therapeutic earnings', but whether this works for any one individual will depend on their particular illness and the cooperation of their doctor. Recent changes to the system of disability benefits in Britain, designed to reduce the number of people claiming, will only leave more of us in the situation where we can neither get appropriate work nor qualify for benefits. Many disabled people in this country, including some of the women in this book, are therefore at risk of living in increasing poverty in the coming years.

Patricia feels that disabled or ill women get a particularly hard deal because their role in the home is not recognized as work. Some women, whose main work is as a housewife or mother, feel especially negative about their reduced energy levels or physical abilities. It is one thing to have an opportunity to re-evaluate a career or paid employment, but housework has to be done and families still have to be cared for; they cannot be so easily re-evaluated or renegotiated!

> Women are expected to have these chronic things, but it's not so terribly important, because they're not the breadwinners. It's considered to be more important to rehabilitate the men than the women. And if they're not rehabilitated then it's not really so much hassle because they've always got women to look after them; but the women look after themselves. They might not be able to do a job of work, a job they were trained for, but they're still expected to manage a home and men are not. My brother-in-law recently had a back injury and he's been offered retraining, a special chair at work and other things. I wouldn't get someone to come and see to the children if I was flat on my back for a week.

Patricia also feels that women are more prone to chronic illnesses because of the kinds of work they do:

> Not many men spend years of their life lifting toddlers up and down stairs so many times in every day. And taking a buggy round the shops is no mean feat. There are different demands on women's bodies, physically and emotionally.

There is no doubt that women and men experience different patterns of health and illness. Although men die earlier, women report much more ill health during their lifetimes and are heavier users of the Health Service (even disregarding the fact that we use it for contraception, pregnancy and other areas of reproductive health).[3] Nevertheless, women's illness is often not taken seriously, quite probably because, as Patricia says, society is too dependent on our unpaid labour to do without it easily. Because this work is unpaid and never costed, society also finds it difficult to replace it. If a woman does become too ill to run the home and look after her children without help, that help is rarely there in the form that she and her family would like. Without resources to support people at home, without recognition of how much work women do, families suffer and children often pick up the work their mother cannot do. The inadequacy and inflexibility of support or care services put pressure on women who are ill not to admit that they need help.

> In the borough that I live in, if you're ill, you can stay at home and get this 24-hour help to come in to cook and do the cleaning, which is really good for HIV-positive women with children. They want to stay at home, they want the children's lives to carry on as normal. But only a few places have that. Some women look for foster carers for their kids, because they don't know how long they'll be around, but there just are not enough foster carers to go around. I can't understand why social services can't recruit appropriate foster carers for different families. But then again it's down to money, they haven't got the money. So there are kids at home with parents who lose their will to live and it's just horrible. That shouldn't be happening.

Increasing reliance on families as carers does not only put more strain on those families, but also leaves disabled women and their children at risk of being stuck in relationships that are physically or emotionally harmful. The threat of abuse is a real, not imaginary one; the lack of accessible housing and support make it even harder for disabled women than for able-bodied women to escape violent partners or parents.

I wanted to leave for a long time, but where can you go when you've got a specially built place which can accommodate a wheelchair and the council says you're housed ... and when you've got young children and there's nowhere to go that's accessible? I wanted to leave particularly because MS accelerates with stress.

*Audrey, a woman with MS*[4]

## 'If you don't contribute, you don't count': fears for the future

As well as our own personal frustrations and the implications for our self-esteem and treatment by others, the ability to work for money or in the home is central to our standard of living and, perhaps, our very survival as we become older or increasingly ill. Women in general lose out over pensions because we often work in lower paid jobs or in casual work, where we do not pay national insurance contributions. We may also work for fewer years than men, leaving to look after the house and children. It is also true nowadays that many families are dependent on a woman's earning power as well as, or instead of, a man's, but the pension and benefits system still reflect traditional assumptions about women's work.

If our paid employment is curtailed by illness, we may fare still worse. We may be at risk of serious poverty if society decides that it wants to spend less on people who are ill, who do not work, who do not pay taxes, who do not contribute. We live in a culture where our rights are not always seen as absolute but as dependent on our behaviour or what we put into society. As Clare says, 'If you don't contribute you don't have rights to all sorts of things.' Grace agrees: 'If you're not the body perfect, fit, physical, then you don't count.' Indeed many of us are fearful as to whether or not we will in future have any rights to decent health care, to independent living and an income.

If we don't count, then how will we prosper in a climate of increasingly harsh competition for shrinking resources? Amidst all the discussion of what work means, we should not forget that primarily it means money, an income on which to live. If we are not allowed, or not able to work, we may not be sure what we will live on, how we will live, or how our health will be looked after.

If anything happens to my partner and I'm on my own ... It worries me that health care might be something to do with how much you earn. Well I earn sod all, so I'm not going to get a very good service. I've got to admit I'm a bit worried, but there's nothing I can do about it, except saving up these 10 pence pieces and hoping to God I can afford a consultant when I get older.

*Harriet*

If they're going to cut social services and they're not giving out enough money for care cover, then I'm going to have to go into a home, which means removal from my own surroundings, from my own property, the loss of my animals. There doesn't seem an awful lot of point in going on if that's the prospect.

*Adele*

## 3

# *Strange Attitudes: Coping with People Coping with Us*

**I**t's hard to go out there as a woman with an illness. You're going out with something. It's not just you and your work and your friends; it's you and your illness, me and sickle cell.

*Paris*

A lot of it is how you approach it yourself, whether you're at ease with it; and there's times when you are and other times when you're not.

*Mary*

Having an illness cannot help but impact on our relationships with the world around us. The sense of our lives being more complicated than those of others or of being easily misunderstood makes social interaction and friendship difficult at times. There is always something extra for other people to take into account, an extra piece of baggage which we carry around with us. Sometimes this takes the physical form of equipment or medication, sometimes it's just a preoccupation in our minds.

Society's failure to value us as disabled women may mean we live with, or have to struggle against, a sense of being second-rate. This will, of course, affect how we feel about other people and our relationships with them. There are endless ways (ranging from the merely irritating to profoundly hurtful) in which the attitudes of others towards us impinge on our lives and make them more difficult than they need be, both practically and emotionally.

## *'Can you catch it?': fear of contamination*

I'm not one of those who like carrying a bright orange sticker around saying 'Beware, I'm unclean!' – but people's attitudes towards you make you think that you are. The attitude of a lot of people is: 'Is it contagious?' And you need to explain to them that no, it's not, and no, you're not a freak.

*Janet*

I think some people, not friends of course, but strangers, tend to think people with physical disabilities have mental disabilities as well.

*Rachel*

Epilepsy is one condition particularly associated with mental impairment or mental illness, partly because the actual fits themselves are frightening for other people. The degree of stigma still attached to epilepsy is undoubtedly related to its perceived connection with mental instability or illness.

Things are changing, but very slowly, and epilepsy is still very much feared because of ignorance. People tend to think that if you're epileptic you're *non compos mentis* as well. It's still something that people feel ashamed of.

*Angela*

A lot of guys think you're daft, you couldn't have a relationship. They stereotype you instead of trying to find out what you're really like as a person.

*Maureen*

Along with fears of mental illness or instability, people have exaggerated fears of contagion or harm from medication, needles or body fluids such as blood. This terror has been exacerbated by the AIDS epidemic, and in some ways is generally in tune with our contemporary, Western obsession with hygiene and the war against germs. But it goes deeper than reason: people are also frightened of touching wheelchairs, crutches or prostheses, as if they may break at the slightest touch or will cause harm. Our equipment and medication represent far more than the plastic, metal or chemicals they are made of. It is disability and difference that people fear or resent, as Bobby knows from the negative and unhelpful reactions she has experienced to various needs resulting from her diabetes and asthma.

> When I had to do a blood sugar count (a test involving pricking a finger to get a drop of blood) at the community centre, two ladies nearly passed out. There isn't anywhere there where you can go to do it in private, and I don't think it should have to be done privately anyway. At one event they didn't want me to do a blood test in the room, so I was shoved in a toilet (not a very clean one either). Several times when I've been out people have refused to let me plug my nebulizer into their electric for 15 minutes. I've had to go into police stations.

## 'People stare a lot': standing out from the crowd

We have already talked about the problems of invisibility, of people not being able to see what is wrong with us. However, given the stigma attached to disability, together with people's fear and negative attitudes towards it, outwardly visible signs of our illness can also be a problem. People find disabled or obviously ill people embarrassing or frightening. We can be made to feel that we are being impolite or unreasonable when we make even quite minor demands, because we have committed the terrible faux pas of reminding them that we are different. Similarly, a woman with sickle-cell anaemia wrote in *Women's Health* newsletter about the persistent and sometimes hostile questioning she encounters at parties when she refuses alcohol.[1] Refusing food or drink marks us out as different, as not part of the crowd.

However, people around us are also fascinated by difference, which can be just as irritating or isolating. Women who use a wheelchair or who walk differently from others, for example, can never just be one of the crowd. They will always stand out and be stared at.

> One of my biggest problems is that because of the curvature of my spine I walk oddly, and people stare a lot. My answer to that is: 'Right, I'm going to dress up – if you're going to look at me, you might as well see something else other than this bent body.'
>
> *Mary*

Once established as different, we seem almost to become public property; people ask questions that are far more personal than anything they would dream of asking someone who was not ill or disabled:

> Strangers accost me in the street, demand to know what I've done to myself, and expect a full medical history. Sometimes it's quite difficult to put them off. I said to one man, 'Oh, it's a long story', and he said, 'It's alright, I've got plenty of time'! I don't have a right to know why they've got a big nose, so why should they know why I'm using a walking stick? People seem to think I'm rude if I won't tell them.
>
> *Eleanor*

Eleanor and other women have also found adults more difficult than children, whose lack of embarrassment, matter-of-fact questions, and acceptance of difference and the world around them are refreshingly easy to deal with:

> Children say, 'What's the matter with your hand, Eleanor?' and I say, 'It's plastic that one', or 'What have you got a walking stick for?' 'Well, I've hurt my leg.' Then they're not interested anymore. That intrusive curiosity, that's an adult thing.
>
> *Eleanor*

> Sometimes children get in your way a bit, or want a go with the crutches – which is a marvellous opportunity to talk to them about it – and all of a sudden their mother's going: 'Mind the lady!' or 'Leave the lady alone!'
>
> *Marlene*

> My sister's daughter, because she sees me a lot and I play with her, when I have a fit, she's not scared because she thinks I'm playing, she's actually laughing.
>
> *Maureen*

Another form of intrusion is when friends, or even chance acquaintances, feel they have a right to comment on the progress of our illness or how we are managing it. Clare has found other people full of unhelpful advice and suggestions about ME, about which so much has been written in the media that everyone thinks they can be an expert:

> ... things like 'Shouldn't you be well enough to go back to work by now?' (I'd be the first to say so if I could!), and telling me to eat natural yogurt every day, or that so-and-so's been made better by a Spiritualist.

Other people's fear and ignorance, their intrusions into the most intimate functions or malfunctions of our bodies, and their often well-meaning but still tiring advice are all powerful reasons for keeping our illness a secret if we have a choice. Many of us can and do choose to 'pass as normal', just as many lesbians and gay men deal with prejudice and discrimination by not being open, or at least being selective about whom they tell about their sexuality. We may also not want to impose on other people (perhaps especially true for those of us who are older and are more likely to have been brought up not to make a fuss about our own needs). There are many things to weigh in the balance: if we tell, people may alter their view of us; if we do not, we have to live with a secret, may have to explain for the first time in an emergency, and may risk people feeling deceived if and when they find out.

Often the visibility of our illness varies at different times or in different situations. We may have a choice as to how much we display signs of weakness or impairment, such as using a wheelchair or a stick to walk with, sitting down or taking medication in public places. Where there is an element of choice, or changeability in our physical state, we are likely to become aware of other people's strong preference for us to look as well as possible and to avoid arousing embarrassment or squeamishness by our 'ill' behaviour. I have been told a number of times that I shouldn't inject insulin in public as many people are frightened of needles. The more 'normal' we look, the more potential conflict there is with people around us, who may fear our stigma becoming attached to them if we are revealed as ill people.

> I don't think my husband liked walking with me when I was using crutches. He used to drive me crazy because he'd either be walking behind me or walking in front. I think he was ashamed of me.
> *Marlene*

Francesca, too, found her ex-boyfriend refusing to go to an art gallery with her when she told him that she'd need to use a wheelchair as the building was so enormous:

He's a lot younger than me and said it wouldn't do his image any good and tried to make a joke out of it.

## *'In my chair or out of it': changing needs and reactions*

People seem to find it particularly hard to grasp that we are not the same all the time, that our physical abilities alter. Some women use a stick or wheelchair for some of the time only and find other people's reactions to them change accordingly.

> The same people treat me completely differently when I'm in my chair and not in it. If I'm in the chair they don't speak to me, only to the person who's with me ...
>
> *Bobby*

Adele has similar problems with neighbours who can't understand the changes in her condition and physical abilities from day to day. She and Bobby both experience the prejudice that exists towards wheelchair-users, as well as the suspicion and confusion people demonstrate towards fluctuating conditions. People prefer us to have a definite identity ('can walk' or 'can't walk') and to stick to it. Apparent inconsistency makes them feel they have been lied to.

> After a few weeks the effect of the chloroquine treatment wears off, so it becomes a big thing for me to do my shopping. I'd love to have a walking stick when I'm like that, but I'd feel too embarrassed. People don't know that when you're not on the treatment you need a walking stick and when you are on it you can be quite active. They would think, 'How come last week she had a stick

and this week she hasn't? She's pulling the wool over our eyes.'

*Shirley*

Since our needs and abilities are not the same every day, we need people to be able to react differently at different times. It would be simple if we could give them one set of rules to follow, but this isn't always possible:

I have a lot more confidence about saying to people, 'OK, I'm deaf. Please look at me when you speak, don't cover your mouth', because that's about basic communication. But those sort of rules are a lot harder with ME, because it's continually changing.

*Clare*

My husband finds it very frustrating because sometimes I'll say, 'I'm alright, I'll do it myself', and other times it'll be, 'For goodness sake, why haven't you done that?' You want the people closest to you to read what you need, and that doesn't happen all the time.

*Mary*

Of course in an ideal world we would like those around us to know what we need without being told – but this would require telepathy! Almost as good would be for people to listen to what we say and react accordingly. In practice, however, people find this hard, partly, I think, because they want some outside corroboration. They want to know for themselves what we can and can't do, rather than have to rely on our word for it. Society has such a terror of malingerers!

An additional concern for some people is that we may not know what is best for us because we are ill. As a result of this, they may not always respond appropriately to our requests for help. Since people react more strongly to things they can see, some of us also attract most sympathy, or hostility, because of an impairment which may be of little importance to us. Paris' feet were dislocated during her birth and so she walks differently from most people. This is not a problem for her, but other people react to it because they can see it. Her sickle-cell anaemia, which is not visible, is definitely a problem at times. Similarly, Eleanor, who decided after her stroke to have her paralysed arm amputated, finds others see her one-handedness as making her disabled, while in reality her life is far more restricted by the pain and exhaustion which are the aftereffects of her stroke.

People also have quite definite perceptions of how serious and disabling various illnesses are, not realizing how much variation there can be in experiences of the same illness.

> One of my neighbours pointed out an article in a magazine about a girl with lupus, a very pretty girl who ran her own business, was able to ride and all sorts of activities. If people read that kind of thing, they think there's not much wrong with you. But it's so varied – some people might only have their skin or joints slightly affected, but they might not have a terribly taxing job, so it's kept under control. And you can meet somebody who's very seriously ill with it who looks quite well.
>
> *Shirley*

The net effect of these oddities and inconsistencies in society's response to illness is that some women get less help than they actually require, while others are treated as weaker and more dependent than they need be. A woman with MS may find herself viewed as tragic and useless, her life virtually over, although she would like to be working. Another woman with ME may have difficulty just getting out of bed, but find her doctor refusing to write sick notes and her employer urging her back to work.

## 'I don't go out much': the search for a social life

Needing help with practical things may make us feel vulnerable in our social life and relations with other people (and how much more so if we know that our need is likely to be doubted?) Illness makes us vulnerable because it means that we are not always in control of ourselves, and this is difficult to manage even with people we know quite well.

> We had a big family get-together. I was having a hypo and I said I wanted some help, but they're all yattering on and I burst into tears because I was really shaky. Then someone did help me, but I don't think they quite understood.
>
> *Tracey*

These kind of experiences are even harder to deal with if we are out in public with people who do not understand at all, and they may make us lose a lot of confidence.

> One time I came out of a shop and I did not know where I was or which way to turn. I just stood there until things came back to me. It's a very bad sensation – you start to panic and feel afraid even to cross the street.
>
> *Joyce*

> When I was pregnant, I had fits all the time. I must have landed up at every hospital in London because, if you have an attack, people invariably call an ambulance. It's not necessary, but they do.
>
> *Angela*

At a meeting for women with diabetes last year, we talked about our fear of 'going hypo' in public and 'making a spectacle of ourselves'. Sometimes people call the police, because they think we are drunk or on drugs.

> Before I get a fit I always get an aura which is a horrible pain, like being battered mentally. But it's good to have a bit of a warning if I'm somewhere that's public because I know to go out of the way, like go in a toilet and try to cool down, so I know I'm not giving everyone a free show.
>
> *Maureen*

It is incredibly unpleasant to be out of control of your body when around people you do not know, and this can make us much less willing to put ourselves in situations we are not used to or do not feel in control of. It may also affect our confidence in meeting new people, whether colleagues, friends or a potential partner, because of their possible reaction to us:

> Sometimes the diabetes takes over me and I get a bit angry, and then it shows and I probably scare people off.
>
> *Tracey*

For some of us, there are practical barriers to having a social life and meeting people. So many forms of social interaction, and places where people meet, are designed for those who are fit, strong and not disabled – for people who can see and hear well, who can cope easily with cigarette smoke, alcohol, music, stairs, uncomfortable seating and so on.

> I don't go out much. I get tired and if it's too dark I can't lip-read easily. Sometimes I find it difficult to concentrate on conversations and every so often I just lose it and have to ask people to say it all over again. So I find meeting new people difficult.
>
> *Clare*

> I don't meet people my own age. I get so tired that I'm only really functioning for a few hours in the middle of the day. Going out for dinner in the evening is out of the question. I tend to meet people who are retired, who do things in the daytime.
>
> *Eleanor*

The amount we may have to explain about our condition to new people may also feel like an enormous hurdle, and it can be difficult finding common ground with people who are very well and energetic. It is hard for other people, both new acquaintances and old, to remember the various things we can and can't do, and hard for us to have to keep reminding them. Sade finds that even her sisters haven't really accepted, for instance, that she can't keep up with them on a shopping expedition. Several women talked about the problems of having different energy levels, or just having to live life at a slower pace than those around them.

> I was always so busy, always out doing things, so all the other people I knew were involved in things as well. When I became ill, I had to give all of that up. My life is very much in the slow lane and other people's are very much in the fast lane. Friends come round and see you, but I think for some of them it's just too difficult.
>
> *Clare*

There may be things which we are perfectly capable of doing, but which we do more slowly than suits our friends or family. Marlene doesn't blame people for not being able to remember what limitations there are on her, but finds it does make it hard to do things together:

> I can't stand a lot. I can go round the market as long as I can sit down now and again or if I keep walking. If I go with a friend they either make me stand because they're looking at something or else they're walking too far. It's

not their fault ... I just can't cope with coping with other people.

*Marlene*

I do enjoy nature and being outside and walking, but I have to be careful how much I do. It's never a hassle to me if I go out on my own. It becomes a hassle because it restricts other people, but only if that's the way they think about it. I have two friends who I walk with where our respective needs are met and it doesn't feel as if my condition is limiting us from having the walk we really want to have.

*Grace*

Going on holiday I worry if it will be a bit of a drag for my husband, because it slows him down when we can't do things. He doesn't really like to go and do them on his own.

*Shirley*

Lesley described how she and other women with radiotherapy injuries feel a burden to family and friends when things like holidays are being planned, because of practical problems with insurance or concerns about whether they will be alright in a foreign country. Shirley got fed up with this constant feeling of being a nuisance to other people:

> Some friends want to meet in town and go walking all over the place and I can't keep up with them, so I prefer to go on my own at my own pace. I've got on better with certain friends, while other people I've dropped or they've dropped me. I suppose I was a bit of a bore to them, so rather than getting upset about it, I'd rather do my own thing with people I feel good with. You don't want to keep feeling put down – you want to shine in your own little way!

Money and food can also be difficult to negotiate in our social life:

The biggest restriction is the food. It's very difficult if you're invited out of the family for a meal, because I inject and then I have to eat before I leave because you can't ask people to change the time they eat for you, and you're sat there while your blood sugar's dropping.

*Bobby*

Friends sometimes forget about my income and standard of living because they're all working with brilliant salaries. And if you've got a colostomy/urostomy, you have to think about when you're going to eat. For instance, going to the theatre, my friend will suggest going for the early cheap menu, but I can't sit through the theatre then because of the noises my colostomy will make, and I don't want to empty my bag in a restaurant toilet. So if I go out to eat, which I really do enjoy, it's got to be later on.

*Lesley*

Some friends and families adapt very easily to these rules and considerations, while others may find it harder to fit in around us or to deal with the fact that they can do different things from us:

One friend doesn't tell me when she does certain things. For instance, if she's going to London for the day for an exhibition she says, 'I know you'd feel so awful that you can't do it.' But I don't really.

*Rachel*

Often decisions are made for us because we're ill. People, especially family, use our illnesses on occasions to suit them and their needs: 'You couldn't go shopping in London all day, that's why I never mentioned it.' Or they don't mind asking me to unload the car, but don't want me looking after the kids.

*Lesley*

The degree of restriction we experience in our social life will vary according to our level of health, our age, and the kind of activities our friends tend to do, as well as their attitudes. Some of us feel little or no restriction, provided we keep to certain rules:

> I can go where I want and do what I want. I think my partner and people around me worry about it more than I do. In my teens and early 20s it was: 'Let's go to the pub then let's go into town, not bother going home.' Then it did make a difference, but if I needed to go home I just did.
>
> *Helen*

The greatest nuisance or difficulty is often the unpredictability of our illness:

> Friends know that I can only make short-term arrangements and sometimes on the day I just can't go. If it's a very bad day, I just go into a corner, I don't see them.
>
> *Rachel*

> Because of extreme exhaustion I can't plan anything, although I can pace myself for big events, with a lot of resting beforehand. So there are limitations, but I carry on.
>
> *Francesca*

## 'Sometimes you feel closed in': more hidden obstacles

Some of the impact on our social life and friendships stems from our feelings of inadequacy in relation to other people. We may feel unable to offer as much hospitality, time or help to other people as we would like:

> I'd have more contact with other women and other families if I didn't find it such hard work. You can't just visit other people all the time. You have to have visits back, which is tiring. It's easier in the summer because I can visit my friend and help her in the garden while the kids play. So they've had a good time and I don't feel we've been a nuisance, and that's great.
>
> *Patricia*

Not only can Joyce not do as much physically for other people as she used to, she also feels that illness has changed her more fundamentally:

> Sometimes you do feel closed in. You can be self-centred sometimes. You have to get hold of yourself and say, 'Oh no, I'm not going down that street with you', because it can bring you to a place where you don't feel like talking, like associating with people. That liveliness, it's cut off, because of your illness. I used to be a person that loved to be with people and I like to do things if I can for people. The lady I call my mum is ill and I like to go and see how she is, but sometimes the way I feel I just can't go, because you have no use to anyone – you just want to sit there in your corner.
>
> *Joyce*

Alternatively, we may have a sense of having more serious concerns to think about than people who are well. While illness does not make us into saints, it may make us think more deeply about some things and, if we have experienced a change from health to illness, then our needs from social contact and friends may also change.

> I just felt like whatever problem they had, it was nothing like mine. When you're working, going out, having relationships, you can have fun, go swimming, have holidays, go dancing. Someone else can be so ill, they can't even sit in the sun because they're allergic to it, they can't write, and they can't even have conversations ...
> *Jessie*

> It's put a bit of a separation between me and some people I know because I can't be bothered with trivial social life, dinner parties, all the jokes they're cracking.
> *Anna*

Anna also talks about the fact that there are jokes and feelings about our experience that we can only share with other people who have the same illness. She has increasingly turned to other HIV-positive women for her main support:

> Friends have been very supportive, no doubt about it. But as the years have gone on, I've wanted to tell them less because there's so much of it all the time. I've got a really good friend who is dying and I think, 'How much can our friends take?' Every time they see me at the moment I'm miserable. How can I tell them everything I'm feeling?

It is always difficult to judge how much you can ask of other people, particularly friends, when you have a problem that is long term. People who have been bereaved often find that while others rally round at the beginning when there is an immediate crisis and practical help to be offered, they find it hard to respond to the very long-term grief which follows. There are only so many times you can reply 'Terrible!' to people's polite enquiry of 'How are you?' For some women, however, it's not so much that they can't talk to their friends, but that their friends feel they can't talk to them:

> If I'm having a hard time physically, family and friends won't make emotional demands on me. They'll think, 'I can't go to her because she's got enough on her plate already.' It drives me mad and it sets limits to relationships. The image of disability that most people have is that you can be brave, courageous, struggling, all those things, but only in terms of your own life. People don't think that you might have things to offer, maybe even that your experience is a useful thing, a learning thing. It can only be a problem.
>
> *Grace*

> The biggest insult is: 'Oh, all the problems you've got and I'm nattering on about my boyfriend problems.' I always say, 'Don't stop telling me, because that's real life. You're ostracizing me and treating me differently if you stop telling me what's really bothering you, what's on your mind.'
>
> *Lesley*

> One of my nicest friends asked me to give her some advice about something and I thought, 'Great! I'm so ill but somebody still thinks that I can give something.'
>
> *Jessie*

So there may be times when we haven't got the energy we would like for other people, but we still want to give whatever we can. When Audre Lorde wrote about feeling isolated with breast cancer, she talked of longing 'to return to the warmth of the fray'[2], and Grace, like Lesley, wants to be involved in other people's lives and problems, because that is real life: 'I'm so much more avid for life now than I've ever been before!'

## 'Who cares and who can't cope': fear, jealousy and other problems

If we develop an illness or become more ill as an adult, people may feel very frightened by the fact that we have changed. Even though the change is not one that we have chosen, there can still be an element of resentment, a fear of being deserted and left behind on the part of those closest to us. We also have to contend with others' fear of death: both the fear that we will die and leave them behind, and the much less readily acknowledged fear of their own death.

> It's really sorted out who really cares about me and who can't cope. There was a great deal of fear when I was first diagnosed, with girlfriends and men friends. They've all said to me since that they absolutely dreaded coming to see me in a cancer hospital, because it had this reputation that if you go in there you don't come out.
> 
> *Lesley*

> I was seeing someone when I first got arthritis. We were working in different cities, but when I was well enough to travel, the first thing I did was to go to see her. I gradually realized, however, that I wasn't welcome and we had a screaming row. She actually said, 'You're no fun anymore, I wanted to go out with someone who was fun. I can't bear to be around you because it makes me think of me being ill, it makes me think of my own death.' All the stuff that most people won't admit to. At the time I found it devastating, I couldn't believe that she had

totally changed her attitude because of me having arthritis. But looking back, it was wonderful honesty, the most honest response I've had from anybody.

*Grace*

Francesca welcomes the changes she has made in her life as a result of becoming ill, but has found that some friends have reacted badly to her illness, at least partly because of this positive aspect of it:

> Some friends who I would have expected to be supportive became quite spiteful when I got a diagnosis, which I found very strange. I think some people feel that you've got an excuse to get out of the rat race and they haven't. Someone said to me that people were jealous because I'm doing things that I enjoy.

> I've got friends who, even though I've got sickle cell and have my problems, they're still jealous of me. A lot of people who have good health take life for granted. One friend, I think, would rather be me and go in hospital than be herself, because she's not happy. She can be quite nasty with me. She just sees that I've got a house, a car, a good job. But she's got all that and doesn't realize it. If I had her health I'd be great!

*Paris*

Maureen has also found that some people seem to resent her getting disability benefits, even though she would rather be working:

> I find that when people hear that I get more benefits than them, because of my illness, they start acting jealous. Like I get more than my sister gets for her and her daughter and I think that's what bothers her. I get more than some people would if they were working, but that's not my fault. I'd rather work than be sat at home doing nowt all day.

If people are in some way jealous, or feel threatened by us saying we have an illness, they may deal with it by deciding not to believe in it, or at least to believe that we are making more of it than we need. As Maureen has found with friends and Sade found with work colleagues, people are very suspicious that we may be using our illnesses to gain some advantage – more benefits, an easier time at work or just extra sympathy.

> I think true friends are very understanding, but people who don't understand, or don't want to understand, feel that you're making a mountain out of a molehill.
>
> *Janet*

Jessie had various problems with other people's reactions to her condition and lost several important relationships. Her partner and others close to her were used to her being in control and perhaps couldn't deal with her now being weak and needing help:

> I lost many close friendships – an ex-lover and another woman whom I thought was one of the people closest in the world to me. I was normally the one who chased after people and made relationships work, but I had to stop having what felt like abusive friendships. They weren't, of course, they were just people having trouble with my situation. Some people were frightened. People felt guilty and then got angry with me. Possibly I was just too needy and they felt as if they would be swamped.

## 'Having to be grateful': getting the help we need

One result of people not being able to deal with our illness is that we may not be able to get help when we need it. Some people are very willing to help, but don't think to ask what it is we actually need. Alternatively they may only want to help in certain ways, so that we may have people around us but still not get what we need.

> What I wanted was someone to take the baby and for me to have a rest. My mother-in-law came round and washed the windows and thought that was what I needed. I don't think people realized quite how knackered I was, because it was a situation that I'd got into so gradually. So people did things that were inappropriate and I was supposed to be grateful and say, 'Oh thank you, you've been such a help!'
>
> *Maggie*

> My husband used to do things for emotional reasons rather than practical ones. He would feel sorry for me and do things that he thought I wanted done. He'd polish all the furniture, but what I wanted him to do was scrub the loo ... People say, 'Oh well, you like to be independent.' How can you be independent when you can't manage? I don't mind people helping me. I don't mind thanking people and I am never rude to people, but it's when you've got to thank them when they're being no use! I thought that when you became ill people rallied round. People you haven't seen in ages turn up in hospital in their best clothes and bring you flowers, but as soon as you're at home and you think you could do with a hand there isn't anybody.
>
> *Marlene*

We are, of course, appreciative of even small amounts of help, when it is the help we need. Woe betide us, however, if we are not grateful! Disability and illness are supposed to make us nicer. Literature is full of cheerful sick people, like Beth in Louisa Alcott's *Little Women*, who are an inspiration to others and brighten the world around them. So besides not wanting to let our friends down, there is also the worry that, if somehow we fail to be ennobled by our experience, to be duly grateful and to make other people feel good, they may in their disappointment decide we are not deserving of help.

> Even close friends think you're being really strong about it and I get quite angry because I feel I've got a right to be fed up and not be able to cope – but you can't because you'll let people down.
>
> *Clare*

Harriet feels that people do want to help but are nervous or don't know what to do. Many people worry about making us upset by talking about it:

> I think people feel unable to help because they don't know how to, so they end up asking daft questions to show an interest. If I go somewhere with my partner, say to a party, when I go and get some food he'll get asked loads of questions while I'm gone. They may not ask me, because they think I might break down or something.

Helen also felt that, although most people want to appear caring, the reality is that few actually have time to think about the needs of disabled people or people who are ill.

> I think most people are fairly ambivalent. We all like to be liked and to be seen to be caring, but if the disability or impairment is going to disturb their lives very dramatically, the only people who are going to stick around you are probably your parents and a partner who

cares very much. For a lot of people, life's hard enough without having to take something else on. Most of us must be guilty of it to some extent. You see somebody who needs to get across the road and you'll help them – but if you're running for the bus, you won't, you think somebody else will do it.

Many of us felt very aware of other people, albeit able-bodied, simply having too much else on their plate to be able to take on board new issues to do with our illness, or to be able to offer practical help. Very few of us or the people we know are untouched by high unemployment, recession, and government policies that have increased poverty, stress and insecurity. We see people around us struggling with children, money worries, job pressures or health problems, which make it hard for them to spare time and energy to help others.

> I think people are suffering these days, certainly in London I notice it, people are really suffering.
> *Jessie*

Some older women among us, or those of us living in working-class communities, look back to a time when there was a greater sense of community, when people helped one another out on a daily basis. Others of us are concerned that the reduction of state resources and the cuts in health and social services put increasing strain on families and individuals. We are all increasingly aware that 'care in the community' in fact means additional unpaid work by women, hardship and poverty for the elderly. It means people with illness living on their own with insufficient support, struggling on with help from friends if they are lucky.

> There are too many people who will look after themselves and think everybody else should do the same. They can't understand that they ought to be responsible in some way for other people. There's none of the community spirit that I would like to see. People don't

expect it because generally they don't get it, and I think things are going to get a lot worse. As generations go on it will be: 'Look after number one', and we'll get more and more elderly people either in care or trying to look after themselves.

*Patricia*

Whether our own experiences have so far been good or bad, we are all aware of there just not being enough spare capacity in society to provide the practical assistance needed by some of us. We may be quite stoical about this, currently feel more worried for others than for ourselves, or may actually be quite frightened for our own future.

## 'I've met some wonderful people': positive discoveries

Despite all these problems, many of us have had lots of support and help from friends, family or neighbours.

> I've been lucky in that I've had intelligent people around me and the friendships were caring friendships – so no problems there.
>
> *Helen*

> My friends were fine, very supportive.
>
> *Jasmin*

> I've got some very good friends who listen and try to help. I get a lot of support from them, and they understand things, like the fact that I can't stay out late.
>
> *Sade*

## Strange Attitudes

It may be our friends more than anyone who refuse to see us as second-rate or tragic disabled people. They may be our touchstone, the people who remind us of who we really are. If we don't have contact with our family or don't live near them, then friends are also likely to be the ones to whom we will turn if we need practical support.

> Friends are very good in terms of offering moral support. I think they still see me as the same person. They're sympathetic and are probably thinking, 'Thank God it's not me!'
>
> *Maggie*

> There are a few close friends I can ask, like if I've fallen down the stairs or I need some shopping done. I have one friend who used to pop in every other day just to make sure I was OK. Another would come and sit while I had a bath because I wouldn't dare have one on my own, in case I had a spasm and drowned.
>
> *Clare*

> People don't know I'm disabled when I'm with my friends because they're covering for me all the time. That's what I want, if I'm in trouble, rescue me, don't bring attention.
>
> *Adele*

Lesley talked about finding out which of her friends really cared about her and which couldn't cope. Certainly illness, in common with a variety of life crises, helps you to find out not only who your friends are, but also much about people's strengths and weaknesses.

> You get left behind and people aren't as important to you as you thought they were. But real friends are still around because they've moved along with you.
>
> *Clare*

If someone has had an illness since childhood, they probably won't have had the same experience of those around them having to respond to change. However, they may consciously or unconsciously have chosen friends who weren't bothered by their condition. They may have learned very early that some people are simply nicer than others:

> When I was growing up I had a lot of friends would bother with me one minute, the next they'd find out I took fits and would sort of push me aside. So rather than have friends like that I don't bother. I've kept myself to myself and just bothered with family and older people, like family friends. When I go out, I mostly go around with older women, like my brother's girlfriend – we're very close. I find young girls, they're scared: 'What if she has a fit?' People a bit older are more understanding and more accepting about it. They don't look at you just in terms of your condition, but as a person.
>
> *Maureen*

We have talked earlier of the ways in which we come to know ourselves better through living with illness. Perhaps we also come to know other people better. Some of us may feel hurt and bitter about people who have let us down. Most of us, however, have also had time to think about and try to understand other people's reactions. We may know that we would not have had any more understanding of illness if it had not happened to us, and that we too don't always do things for other people as perhaps we should. We are very appreciative of the people who are good to us and good for us, but hopefully, over the years, also acquire some compassion, or at least tolerance, towards those who have been able to offer less. There are so many positive discoveries to be made about people and our relationships with them:

> I've got my friend who knows me from school, who'll be there all my life and see me through thick and thin. If

I had perfectly good health, I probably wouldn't know which ones really cared about me. I go into hospital and I know who comes to my bedside. I know they've brought flowers and they're thinking about me. I know one of my friends doesn't rest until I come out of hospital.

*Paris*

... the absolute wonder and therapeutic value of hugs and physical closeness, not just when you're in pain, but generally I'm much more aware of the need and the value of close contact with people.

*Grace*

Finally, of course, there is the fact that we meet different people as a result of living with an illness, people we might not have met if we were healthy. Many disabled people have found their whole perspective on life change, not just through their own experience, but through meeting other disabled people. We may learn a lot from people who have been ill for longer than us, or we may make special bonds with people who, like us, view life differently and have had to think about it harder than others. And, just as illness and change may expose us to the worst of other people's weaknesses or malice, so too we may see some of the best of human behaviour:

You know, my life would have been very different if I hadn't had an illness. But it's also been quite rewarding in some ways, from a positive side. I've met some wonderful people, interesting people.

*Mary*

I have made friends through being disabled. I met a guy at the art workshop who is a facilitator. I didn't know what a facilitator was and this fellow turned up to help me. On the first day I thought it was going to be like with my husband – I was going to have to explain what I wanted and we'd have an argument about why I wanted it. But no, he just did what I wanted, made no helpful suggestions, was completely non-judgmental and it turned out exactly how I wanted. Isn't that absolutely wonderful what he did for me? So that's a wonderful person I've met who I wouldn't have met otherwise.

*Marlene*

# 4

# *Not a Real Woman?: Love, Sex and Families*

**I** always had this idea that I'd never get married and never have children. I just wanted to be an independent person all my life, do my own thing. Suddenly I'm not – but it's nothing to do with having kids or living with my partner. It's to do with this illness; suddenly I can't do everything for myself.

*Harriet*

I can't have sexual intercourse, can't have children. I look alright and men still try and chat me up, and I think, 'Jesus, if only they knew!' You are emotionally and mentally stripped of your womanhood. You've had that many prods and pokes down there that you no longer feel sexual at all.

*Lesley*

There's this all-round woman image: somebody who works out and has a job, is kind and nice and well-groomed as well. I'm having to get used to being a different shape, a slightly older, heavier shape. I keep thinking I should be able to exercise and firm up, but physically I can't do very much.

*Francesca*

We each have our own idea of what it means to be a woman, formed in line with, and in opposition to, the ideas of womanhood offered to us by society. To be a woman may mean to be pretty, sexy, strong, nurturing, independent – all qualities that can be undermined or changed for us by illness or disability. The world of work is one area where conflicts and questions arise about the nature, as well as the status, of women. However, women are so strongly identified with the family and with sex and children, that it is perhaps here, in our closest relationships, that the greatest or most negative impact of illness can be seen.

## 'The sex side of things': physical and emotional difficulties

Sexuality is immensely complicated, individual, and often regarded as too private to talk about, even for 'normal' people with their normal bodies. Only good-looking people are supposed to have sex; even the idea of fat or old people having sex makes others uncomfortable and so becomes something to joke about. The sexuality of disabled women is considered still more taboo, since it is not even supposed to exist.

As women we are defined as sexual beings. The outside world defines and judges us both as a potential object of male desire and according to how much we can satisfy that desire. At its most basic, this is about whether we consent to and are able to have ordinary sexual intercourse. Some women with radiotherapy injuries have been too badly damaged for vaginal penetration to be pleasurable or even possible. This makes them unthinkable as a sexual partner for many, probably most men, although as Lesley says, 'You can do other things in bed.' When Patricia consulted her doctor about her loss of desire for sex (which turned out to be caused by the medication she was on), he asked with considerable concern if this meant that she was refusing to 'oblige' her husband, which would be 'very naughty'. Luckily she sought advice from another doctor and was able to come off the medication, but, as she says:

> It was an awful time in our relationship. If he wasn't the man he is, we wouldn't have survived at all. There's not many men as patient as he is.

Sex is of course a huge issue for women with HIV, as the following extracts from Positively Women's survey show. Some women may have found it an opportunity to think about their sexual relationships or practice and what they want from it, but fear looms very large, both for the women themselves and their partners:

> I'm more aware of what I want sexually.

> It's not spontaneous anymore.

> I am afraid of starting a relationship with a man because of my HIV status. I don't want rejection or abuse.

> Seeing my partner with a condom reminds me I'm HIV positive.

> I try to assert the use of condoms but my partner will not take me seriously.

> We no longer have sex.[1]

The actual importance of sex in our relationships will of course vary among us. However, if we live with a partner, then the relationship is identified as a sexual one, so whether or not sex is something we do together is significant. It is one of the main ways in which we express our closeness and continued desire to be together. Women, as well as men, are now encouraged to have high expectations of themselves and their partners in a sexual relationship. So it matters if we are no longer able to have sex, no longer want sex, or if our sexual activity is limited in any way by our illness or condition.

> My feelings for him have diminished a lot, partly because of the difficulty of sex together. I go to bed at nine or ten when he's going out to the pub. But it's not just my tiredness; he's a much more physical person than I am and bedroom gymnastics have gone out the window because the cancer was in my spine and I mustn't jerk it. We've found a way or two round it, but it's difficult, so I'm quite content to go to sleep or pretend to be asleep when he comes home. It happens in a lot of marriages, but it's more important somehow because I'm rejecting him.
> *Woman at a cancer support group*

There are a whole range of practical limitations on our sexual activity caused by our particular conditions. Some are reasonably obvious, such as a lack of mobility or suppleness, pain and stiffness:

> In terms of sexual practice, it's been quite difficult. Part of lesbian culture is having quite an active sexuality. There are challenges to that. There are celibate lesbians, but it's still focused on that. It is the most difficult area of relationships to talk about, especially initially when you're getting together with someone – you don't want to spend all the time talking about what you can't do. I haven't had a partner who's been particularly sensitive, who's thought about what my condition is and how that might relate to what we do in bed. The responsibility has been left with me. I've been in situations where I'm in pain and then someone's saying, 'Well, why didn't you tell me?'
> *Grace*

## Not a Real Woman?

In a sexual relationship I don't develop a headache, I develop backache. After a few hours of rolling in the hay I'm not going to be very well for a few days. It doesn't rule my sex life, but the strain on the back is incredible and if I can't or don't feel like performing later on during the week then I don't. Whoever is with me would have to accept that.

*Adele*

When I was first diagnosed with diabetes, I felt it would be an enormous turn-off for a partner to witness me sticking a needle in myself last thing at night. Sexuality is not just about what we can and cannot do in bed, but also about feeling good about ourselves and our bodies. Illness can therefore have a considerable effect on our sexual confidence. Women with colostomy bags, for example, are likely to feel worried about smell or their bags bursting in the night if they are sleeping with someone. In fact just wearing incontinence pads and having one or two bags attached to your body does not make you feel very sexy. It also affects what clothes you can wear, which for some of us may play an important part in how we express our sexuality:

You have to wear things that won't show your bag, so it can't be anything slinky or clingy.

*Lesley*

Women I talked to at a cancer support group said that while some men leave partners who have had a mastectomy, many women themselves reject sex and their partners because they no longer feel confident about their one-breasted bodies – bodies that no longer match up to the idealized versions we all see portrayed everywhere:

I don't like him to see me; there's no way I'll let him in the bathroom with me anymore.

> My hubby was wonderful. I wouldn't let him see my body, I really felt ashamed. But he coaxed me, said, 'Come on, let me have a look.' So now I'm not bothered.

Breast cancer is one of the diseases women fear most, perhaps because of the threatened loss of a breast, the symbol of femininity with which our culture is so fixated. Audre Lorde talks about the irony of women who have had mastectomies being encouraged, even bullied into concealing this fact by wearing prostheses or having potentially dangerous breast implants, so as to appear still 'normal', still desirable women. When she visited her breast surgeon's office for a follow-up appointment, she was reprimanded for not wearing a prosthesis because it lowered the morale of the office!

> Here we were, in the offices of one of the top breast cancer surgeons in New York City. Every woman there either had a breast removed, might have to have a breast removed, or was afraid of having to have a breast removed. And every woman there could have used a reminder that having one breast did not mean her life was over, nor that she was less a woman, nor that she was condemned to the use of a placebo in order to feel good about herself and the way she looked.[2]

Our illness may also make us put on weight or lose weight, or can cause other changes to our bodies which make them no longer feel our own. Another problem for some of us is that our partners may have to help at times with things such as medication, pain relief or cleaning ourselves, which we may feel prevents them from being able to see us as sexy or exciting.

> I put on weight and my face was very puffy. I felt very unattractive and didn't feel that my partner would be attracted to me sexually. It made me feel a different person. This condition reduces your sex drive anyway

and I'd just had a baby and was still sore. The sex side of things was very difficult for a while.

*Maggie*

I joke with him, 'When you got married you didn't think you'd be rubbing cream into your wife's limbs in bed!' It does affect your personal life – energy levels, cramp and positions you have to adopt.

*Patricia*

I went to see the film *Pretty Woman* when it first came out. She was in the bath while he was talking to her and then walking around without clothes on and I thought, 'I couldn't do that.'

*Lesley*

Sex and sexuality are complicated for women by the inequality of heterosexual relationships, so strongly ingrained in our society that it also impacts on sexual relationships between women. The culture we live in does not respect women's bodily autonomy. So much of the time the needs or rights of others, in particular men or babies, are seen to take priority over our own. Many of us, therefore, have only a precarious sense of control over what happens to our bodies, and those who have experienced sexual abuse or assault are likely to feel especially powerless in the act of sex. We may feel that illness in itself reduces our control over our own body, or that our control is threatened because we are physically weaker than our partner.

> Being a woman and not having physical strength has connections for me with being a survivor of child sexual abuse, because it's like being a child with an adult again. In the past, I have had a tendency to play out that role and to believe that I don't have rights to express what I want in a sexual relationship. I only started to deal with it when I became disabled, because being in a situation that echoes the original one is insupportable. I have a choice

– either to stay celibate and safe for the rest of my life because it's too risky to deal with all that, or to deal with it in the hope of having a relationship based on communication and equality.

*Grace*

Alternatively, illness may push us into taking more control over our sexual life and communicating our needs more clearly. Physical difficulty or inequality means that we can't afford to be as passive or accepting as women often are in relation to sex and relationships. Partners who cannot respect what we need and want are indeed insupportable, but we may also feel guilty and inadequate towards those partners who do understand and who do put their own needs second to ours.

Our physical nature and physical affection are not only expressed through sex itself, of course, but in all sorts of contact with partners. Illness can interfere here too in a myriad of different ways.

You're not always well enough for the physical side of things and often you hurt if somebody touches you. I feel sorry for my husband because he's got a lot to put up with. You're not always affectionate, because even a hug sometimes hurts you.

*Shirley*

So, as with other aspects of our social life, illness may simply make us less confident, free, spontaneous and giving than we would like to be. Not only does this set up feelings of guilt and inequality in our existing relationships, but it is also a substantial barrier to forming new relationships.

## 'A right liability': problems for new partners

As mentioned in Chapter 3, we cannot fail to be aware that there are issues for potential partners to take on board about which, if they are well and able-bodied, they may be prejudiced or just uncertain and frightened.

> I think with potential relationships the person can be not exactly put off, but they can be wary. Somebody I was having a flirt with the other day said to me, 'God, you're a right liability! You never know if your legs are going to give way or if you're going to throw up!' You can take it as a joke, but it does have to be considered.
>
> *Francesca*

> Before I got married I was almost engaged to somebody. I had an attack and that was it, he walked off. He let it be known that he wasn't going out with a girl who had epilepsy. Things were very different then, we're going back a few years.
>
> *Angela*

Paris says that having sickle-cell anaemia forces a decision early on in a relationship as to how serious it is:

> If my partner and I decide to get married, he's not marrying a healthy person, he's marrying someone who's got an illness and you have to talk about what would happen if you died: would I like him to go and marry somebody else, and what would happen to our children? I prefer to tell someone straight away, rather than risk getting involved and then finding out they can't handle it. There's only been my current partner and one other boy who've stuck by me. It must be difficult for them really.

She and Maureen have both experienced rejections from men who had seemed to be interested but who fled when they found out about their conditions. Epilepsy, as already mentioned, arouses fears of mental impairment, and with sickle-cell anaemia there is fear about it being passed on to children. They both feel clear that people have to accept them with their illness or not at all and, as Paris says, if men can't cope then 'they're not worth knowing'.

> I've not had sex yet because I have problems with men accepting my illness. I get people asking if I'm gay, stuff like that, and my sister saying I'm always going to be a virgin. It's just that I ain't losing it overnight to just anybody. I know a lot of girls who are in sexual relationships, so sometimes I feel a bit out of place. I won't have sex for the sake of being one of the girls. But I worry whether I'll meet somebody and have a proper family relationship.
>
> *Maureen*

All these factors make it hard not only to meet new partners, but also to feel confidence and trust in the possibility of a relationship. We may have learned to be fairly self-sufficient and do not want to expose ourselves to other people's muddled emotions or inability to cope with illness or disability.

> I've had relationships since I've been ill. Some have been catastrophic, really bad! I think I would be very wary about getting into another relationship. I feel there have to be sort of ground rules. For it to work somebody has to understand a lot.
>
> *Clare*

> I don't want somebody holding me up and saying, 'Well, I think you should be doing better than that', or 'You're laying it on thick.' I used to justify how I was to people – well, the hell with that. But I am terrified of relationships

because they'll see me when I'm very ill and when I'm distraught because of the pain, and all the bruises on my bum from the injections. When I'm in pain I don't want anybody near me, as all my barriers go down and I just sit here all miserable and mardy.

*Adele*

Some women are quite happy not to be in relationships, or are at least resigned to it at this stage of their lives. Marlene had the same anxieties as many other women about whether having arthritis would make it difficult to have relationships, but in fact found that it didn't create problems:

I have had a couple of men friends since my husband died and I thought, 'How am I going to cope with this?' But the man I met was very kind, a mature, nice man and it [arthritis] didn't really make any difference to our relationship. It was really smashing while it lasted, and then I met another chap and that was nice. A woman in my position and my age, an elderly widow, well I might have met two more men anyway, or I might not. But still having arthritis I did meet them.

I'm glad sometimes that I'm on my own, because if I had a husband here who don't understand, I don't know what would happen. He would come in and there would be no food because I'm not in the mood for that, or whatever ... I have met up with so many disappointments, I could write a book! I don't bother with men now. If you're sitting and grudging over not having a partner, well, you're in trouble. If you know you want something out of the shop but you can't go there and get it, will you sit and fret about it? There's no point in sitting and fretting because it makes you ill.

*Joyce*

## 'A lovely wife?': men's attitudes to women

Many of us who do have relationships with men identify sexist attitudes and views of women, rather than our illness itself, as the major problem both in starting new relationships and having relationships which are supportive and good for us. In particular many of us have had problems with men's attitudes towards women and towards disability, and other problems have arisen because of differing views as to how relationships work and about male and female roles within them. For example, our image-conscious society defines beauty and attractiveness in very narrow terms, and what a woman looks like determines not only her own status but also that of the man who 'owns' her.

> It's almost like it reflects badly on them [if we are disabled]. Women are expected to be a status symbol, aesthetically and sexually.
> *Francesca*

Men's expectation that a woman with an illness needs looking after may also make them frightened of or threatened by us. Many men assume that women generally are weak and that we are even weaker – and more dependent – because of our illness.

> I think men are scared of being emotionally pressured by a woman who's disabled or sick as well. They always assume anyway that a woman is far more interested in them than they are in the woman, that a woman is going to be clingy and going to want something more from them than they're prepared to give.
> *Francesca*

> Men tend either to treat me as bone china (and then when I need them to treat me like bone china they walk

away) or see me as a challenge – I'm not really ill, I'm only doing that to trap them, or I can cope with my illness because I'm so strong, so also I'm a challenge. So what they want to do is break me down and make me subjected and submissive and sub-anything.

*Adele*

Men's fear of being trapped by a dependent, 'sickly' woman would seem to have more to do with their own general worries about women and relationships than with women's actual expectations of them. Most of us not in a relationship would ideally like to be in one, but none of us are looking for a man, or woman, to look after us. More often we are in fact afraid of losing our independence if we enter into a new relationship. For this reason, some of us may prefer to keep sexual relationships casual:

I had a relationship about a year ago which failed miserably. I involved him very much in my life and he failed me, so the attitude now is that all men are good for is bed. I have a very low opinion of men, very low. With this little fling I had recently, I was happy not to get involved. It came as a shock to him though, when I flung him out in the morning!

*Adele*

However, this idea that we both need looking after ourselves and are less capable than 'normal' women of caring for others is very common. It may not only be a reason for men to be wary of entering into a relationship, but also for their families to see us as less than ideal partners:

When we told his mum about my illness it didn't go down at all well. It was the worst mistake of my life. She told him she didn't want him to be looking after me for the rest of his life (because that's what happened in her life), and she didn't want her grandchildren getting this illness (she didn't understand that bit of it). He's from a different background than me and his mum and dad were probably expecting this girl with a degree, white, middle class, going to be a lovely wife. But we live in the real world and it didn't happen. I know I'm not the healthiest person in the world, but I have a lot to offer and I wish she'd just sit down and talk to me.

*Paris*

As we all know, women are generally supposed to be the carers in relationships with men and with children. Some men feel profoundly undermined and threatened by the possibility of having to take on a caring role in relation to their woman partner or children. They may also resent the fact that they are not getting cared for enough themselves. A wife or mother with a chronic illness presents a long-term challenge to traditional divisions of labour and roles within the home, which some men are simply unable or unwilling to accept. Jessie's ex-partner refused to believe in the seriousness of her illness, seeing it as 'a plot to get out of having children with him'! However, his unwillingness to look after her was also partly rooted in differences in class and power:

> I'm from a middle-class background and usually someone who is quite in control and has a lot of power. My ex-partner is working class and I know that me asking for help made him feel like a servant, even when I was too weak to lift up my hand to brush my hair.

Mary, too, found that her first husband dealt with her illness and their children's health problems by simply denying their existence:

> He found it very difficult to cope with illness. He was very unsupportive. He just used to shut his eyes and pretend I wasn't ill and I coped with the children.

> My husband doesn't understand why I get upset about it. I don't talk to him as much as I did; it's the feeling that he

might not understand, that's what stops me, because it will hurt me more then.

*Kabita*

We have already looked at how men deal with their own illness differently from women. They also deal with the illness of others differently. A woman at a cancer support group described how she had collected leaflets and books for her husband to read. She did this partly because she wanted him to know more so that he could support her, but also because she felt it would help him if he understood about the disease and treatments. His response, however, was: 'It's enough that you've got cancer without me having to read about it as well.'

Those close to us may well deny the seriousness of our illness, or at least not want to know too much about it, because they fear both our death and their own; and perhaps men are more likely to do this than women. In addition, however, there is always pressure for women's illness not to take too great a priority in a relationship or household.

For example, if it was my husband [who had diabetes], the whole family would be having to eat the same food [as him] now, wouldn't they? Because he's not well, I am not going to make any sweets in the house. Men don't think that way. He will still buy sweets I like and say, 'Oh, have one, it doesn't matter.' He's a doctor as well! If you are a woman, you think you should stop him from eating sweets, or whatever restrictions there are, if he is ill.

*Kabita*

Several of us talked about the fact that men's fear of having to care for someone who is ill seemed particularly ridiculous since in reality women tend to do much more caring for men than the other way around:

I suspect a lot more disabled men get looked after by partners of whatever gender than vice versa.

*Francesca*

> There are all these men who are leaving their wives with radiotherapy illness; the women would stay, there'd be no two ways about it. The women would stay, but the men don't.
>
> *Lesley*

> You won't see many disabled or ill women sitting in the pub chatting and having a nice sociable time because they're not able to work – they've still got to do the shopping and the housework.
>
> *Patricia*

One question in my mind when I started this book was whether or not women in lesbian relationships had an easier time of it than those of us who live with men, and whether in general women are more sympathetic and supportive in their response to illness.

> I haven't had a girlfriend for a couple of years, but the relationship is totally different. I was trapped in bed one day and my girlfriend brought all my stuff upstairs and then came and sat with me. She read and we had the music on and it was great. With a recent boyfriend, however, though he also brought my stuff up when I was ill, he brought it up one item at a time. I had to keep asking for things, it was so begrudging. Then he went off and tinkered with his car and sat downstairs and didn't come up again. It was a totally different attitude. So I think there's a comradeship between women that doesn't exist with men. I tend to bring out that need to protect (in women) that I don't find in men.
>
> *Adele*

Not all women are natural carers, however, and some women have experienced rejection by women partners or friends, which has been particularly devastating because less expected. Many women, whether or not they call themselves feminists, have low expectations of men and very high ones of women. We may have assumed that women friends or lovers would handle our illness well and then have been very let down when they didn't. Also, just as in heterosexual relationships, both real, physical differences and socially constructed roles can make it hard to negotiate equality in lesbian relationships:

> I don't in any sense like to feel that I'm being looked after, and a couple of times I've nearly got involved with someone where that was the attraction, they were looking for someone to look after and I was a pretty good candidate. Women are much better at the looking after side of relationships. But when you're disabled that means you can end up being mothered in a way that's inappropriate in a sexual relationship. I found that I was doing most of the cooking and my partner was doing most of the physical stuff. It makes you feel like you're role-playing, and certainly the perception of family and friends was that my partner was the active one and I was the homemaker. I find it extraordinary that I could get into that situation, because it's so far from how I think about myself. Yet because of the disability, it's been how things work out sometimes.
>
> *Grace*

## 'I do feel guilty': letting people down

Perhaps the hardest thing to deal with in any relationship is inequality or difference, especially between men and women. Some kinds of inequality are at least in theory open to negotiation or change (such as in earning power or the division of labour), whereas our physical needs or limitations may be less adaptable. The problems seem to be greatest for those of us who are having to get used to a change or where there is most obvious difference between us and our partners. Women who are or have been in relationships with other disabled people feel they understand more of our experience than an able-bodied partner would. There is also a greater sense of equality in the relationship than is felt by women with non-disabled partners:

> My current partner has a disability which in a lot of ways I think is worse than mine. He's deaf, and deafness is something that's laughed at, so he has that understanding.
>
> *Helen*

> The relationship I had before was with another disabled woman. In some ways that was easier because I didn't have to explain lots of things.
>
> *Clare*

Mary's partner is quite a few years older than her:

> My second husband is older. He's slowed down quite a lot. He actually said when we first decided that we were going to live together, 'Because you're ill and you've slowed down, that's fine, we can work it together.'

Such relationships avoid the sense of indebtedness and dependency that is common within many of our relationships. One of the principal ways in which we may feel inadequate or guilty towards our partners (as with other family and friends) is when we are unable to keep up with their level of activity:

> It was really difficult trying to have a relationship with somebody quite energetic who wanted to do things, when you're someone who can't think further than, 'How am I going to get the energy to go to the toilet and get back and go to sleep?' In some ways you feel you're

missing out, and you feel guilty that your lover's missing out.

*Clare*

Our partners may take on a disproportionate share of household tasks, or at least, if they are men, more than most men do. Most of us feel that men should be doing work in the house, but within our individual relationships we may have a sense that they do more than is fair if they are the main breadwinner as well. Alternatively, we may just feel uneasy or unhappy that the situation has come about through the necessity of our illness, rather than as a result of thought and negotiation. Our sense of guilt at not fulfilling our 'proper' female role is sometimes so great that we may minimize how much we actually do. However it is also true that, while our partner may be the person we most resent at times, we also have a more intense awareness of their physical and mental state than we do of anyone else bar ourselves or our children. We know when they are tired and overworked, and our feelings of guilt towards them start from the same place as empathy and compassion. It is because we love them and want the best for them that we regret it if our physical state puts extra work onto them.

> He's so caring. We've been married 40 years. He must get fed up sometimes. I do pay someone to help me dress, not every day, but so he doesn't have to do it always. I don't want him to spend his retirement looking after me.
>
> *Rachel*

I can't imagine anything worse than walking in after a full day's manual work to somebody sat at the table saying, 'I'm so weary, how am I going to finish cooking the tea and washing up?' He must feel awful sometimes walking in to that. He never says that he does. It makes you feel a right heel; sometimes I could thump him, he's so good. I'd feel better sometimes if he wasn't, but I do thank God that he is. He'll tire himself out to do things for me. I'd like that to change. I wouldn't feel guilty if I was able, I'd say he should take his turn. But I do feel guilty about him doing these things because I'm too tired or unable.

*Patricia*

I think most men should be more equal. My partner is quite fit so he does the stairs and things I can't really manage, but then I think he works too hard, so I feel I'm putting on him a bit.

*Shirley*

We may also feel regret or guilt at having brought pain and worry into our partner's life. A couple of women at a cancer support group said they felt guilty for having had cancer or had a mastectomy, and one reason for coming to the group was to take some of the emotional load off their partner:

My husband's mother died of cancer when he was 12, and I felt like I had let him down. I thought, 'Oh God, he's had enough, he doesn't want this.'

I think it was a really difficult period for my partner. I did lean on him very heavily and he had to hide how he felt a lot of the time. It must have changed how he sees me because he's seen me at my most vulnerable and pathetic. I think he just wishes I was the same as before.

*Maggie*

My partner has said it was really hard for him to admit sometimes that I was too tired to do things, and to accept that I was quite different to how I was when we met.

*Jasmin*

We may feel guilty simply about the fact of having changed – that our partners have ended up with a different person or a different relationship to the one they originally thought they were getting.

> I get quite upset about that because I feel he's been sold a pig in a poke. You see other women at 43 who are still very active and full of life.
>
> *Patricia*

## 'Mum treats me like I'm two years old': restrictions in the family

It is not only our partners, however, who have to deal with the fact that we have changed. So too do our parents and other family members, who may find it especially hard since they have known us for so long. The closer people are to us, the more they may have to fear from us changing, and of course the more frightened they will also be about our survival. Sade's brother died of sickle-cell anaemia in his teens and so when she became ill her parents were terrified that she too might die. Maggie's father and brothers were also frightened by her diagnosis of an underactive thyroid because they had seen her mother die of thyroid-related causes:

> I felt I had to protect them when it was diagnosed. I'd always given this impression of toughness and of being independent and self-motivated. I think it came as a great shock to my dad and brothers to realize that I was vulnerable; they'd never seen me being such a wretch before.

> Every time I go into hospital, I look at my mum and see her sad face and it makes me cry. Even if I'm in terrible pain and I think it's the end, I always tell her, 'I'll live for you', and that makes her happy. I feel very guilty towards

my mum and dad because I know they're in pain to see me lying there when they can't do anything. My dad hates going to hospitals.

*Paris*

Families are complicated groups and illness on the part of one member may have a considerable impact on everyone else in the family. However, because it is an obvious, tangible problem, our illness may get blamed for things which are in fact nothing to do with it; and the relationships that illness affects are affected by many other emotions and issues.

It had a terrible impact on my parents. My father has developed a heart condition and I know that is because of what he's been through with me being so ill. There's been other funny things that have gone on, like my sister feeling guilty because she's well, and my parents' drinking problem has been blamed on my illness.

*Lesley*

The way we was brought up, I think I've turned out better for it than my sister in the end. My parents expected her to become somebody and do things with her life, and they expected me to be someone dependent – but it meant she was never pushed or had to try hard. And now she's had two little ones and ended up going back home, and I think she's jealous of me in some ways. When we were young she helped me a lot, although she's younger than me, because she was always there when I had fits; one time she actually saved my life.

*Maureen*

I'm the oldest and when I was younger I used to protect my sister, but now she's the one that looks after me. It's good.

*Paris*

If you have grown up with your illness, its role within your family may be especially complex. Although there may not be a change from health to illness, the family will still have to deal with change as you grow older and make your own decisions as to how you deal with illness. Most of us experience the families we grew up in as sources of strength and security, as well as restriction and guilt. For several women, however, the family was the place where they were most disbelieved and damaged. As I have already mentioned, Mary's family had little attention to spare for her because of other problems, and Adele's mother was violent and all her family have consistently refused to believe in her disability.

If we did have a bad relationship with parents then the possibility of being dependent on them is particularly frightening:

> When I had the stroke they saw themselves as the devoted parents of a disabled daughter. They were going to keep me in a wheelchair, feed, dress and bath me and get a bit of glory that way. My father was not a bit pleased when he found out I wasn't going to stay in a wheelchair and that I was going to drive a car. He did his best to stop me getting a car.
> 
> *Eleanor*

Some of us have parents who, while not absolutely controlling, may still expect us to take on more of an 'ill' or dependent role than we wish to:

> Family are far more protective. Because you're ill and perhaps because you're not married, they feel they've got an automatic right over your life. Everybody nearly died that I was staying here and not moving home, because that's what they all thought I should do. Even my little nephew said, 'We'll clear out the attic for you', like something out of *Psycho*! My family don't think any man would want me now, which doesn't help my self-worth at all.
> 
> *Lesley*

In the most loving and supportive family, it is still hard for us to get acknowledgement of changes in our lives and of our ability to be independent and look after ourselves. In the family, we are essentially supposed to remain the same person we were as a child, with the same relationships to other people in that group. Change is difficult for us as well as for them. Harriet feels sad that, just as her parents are getting to the age when they might need help themselves, her diagnosis of MS means they have had to start worrying about her again:

> You have this child and you look after her and finally she's off your hands – she's got a fella and a family. Then suddenly, because she's not well, you get all the worry back.

Even where our parents are not actually trying to take over, we may feel irritated that they don't allow us to make our own decisions about our health or illness. It is difficult at times sorting out those decisions for ourselves, and still more difficult when we have to explain or account for them to other people, or even when we just have to worry about them worrying.

> The biggest problem, in the nicest possible way, is my mother. She's in her 80s now and is a very caring person, but she does tend to wrap me in cotton wool. I'm quite grateful that she's 200 odd miles away because I think if she saw the things I do some days she'd have 40 fits. I was very ill one time when I was with her and they didn't know whether I would pull through. It must have been a horrendous experience for her. I think still to this day the memory lingers on.
>
> *Janet*

It's difficult coming from a Nigerian background but being born here – my parents don't think the same as I do about illness. They say, 'Make sure you're well-covered up', 'Take your penicillin every day', even more so now that I've been getting ill a lot more often than when I was young. It's always my fault if I get ill – it's because I went out for a meal, or went on holiday or didn't dress up warmly. They think I mean to be ill. That makes me sad.

*Paris*

When they were here, they saw my lifestyle and didn't like it. They thought I should regularize my life more. I should take more rest. I should go to bed early, I should not eat the biscuits the way I used to. Then the diabetes would be controlled better.

*Kabita*

Parents and partners can sometimes seem to be the people who are hardest on us and blame us most for our illness. Because they care about us and are afraid, they want more than anyone to believe that we can stay well if we do the right things. They may be disproportionately angry with us if we make decisions which differ from the medical advice we get, or don't fit with their own ideas about good health. Parents may also want more from us than we can manage. They may be worried or sympathetic, but still find it hard to accept that we can't do things, or that we are less strong than them even though they are older.

They're a bit demanding really, with the shopping and housework and things. They forget and I have to remind them that I can only do so much. I've tried to explain but I can't really get through to them sometimes.

*Sade*

My parents are very sympathetic and supportive, but they don't always seem to understand that you can't go to visit them every weekend, that you get tired.

*Shirley*

It can also be extremely hard to negotiate changes in their routine when we visit parents or other family. Tracey has had diabetes since the age of 18 months and is now 23. She lives on her own and manages her diabetes herself, but still finds that:

> My mum treats me like I'm two years old, as if I can't look after myself. I have problems when I go to stay with her, because she eats much earlier than I do, which makes the diabetes difficult to control.

Different generations invariably have different beliefs and views about normal daily routines, such as the right food to eat and when to eat it, for example. Differences between us and our parents can often represent these differences between generations: our new ideas, their resistance to change. Requests from us about eating different food or some other change of routine, even if these are for the good of our health, may therefore seem like a challenge or criticism of their way of life. In particular, requests or demands relating to food can also bring up deep-seated resistance to the idea of children being 'fussy' about food. Other areas of difference may be to do with different politics or perspectives on the world, and it can be hard when parents see us very differently from how we see ourselves, as Clare has found:

> It's been quite difficult with my mum. She finds it harder me being deaf than having ME; whereas I don't have any problems with being deaf, but the ME has affected everything.

It is, of course, not only parents and partners who worry about us or judge our behaviour, but also our children, especially as they grow older, and the wider family around us. Mary and Bobby both felt that it is often the people closest to us who are most restrictive and who prevent us doing things we would like to do. In Mary's case, it is children and old friends who have not really adjusted to the fact that she is less incapacitated and can be more active since having hip replacement operations:

> A lot of people down here do accept me for what I am, but if I go home to Scotland, I have to step into another role and allow them to help me, even though I find that very hard and frustrating. I've got more able to do things now, but I have to slip back into that relationship for their sake more than for mine. My daughter is the same all the time on the phone: 'Are you sure you can do this?'
>
> People say, 'Slow down', but I know my own limitations. If I'm going too fast then I'll slow down myself. Let me live. Don't take that away! I'm never allowed out on my own, not allowed out in supermarkets. The children say, 'No, mum, you can't do this, you can't do that' – so I find that an ongoing battle.
>
> Bobby

The wider family is also a place where we can feel our needs are ignored. A family is a group within which no one individual's needs are supposed to dominate. This can mean, even if our immediate family are generally supportive, that in larger gatherings we are expected to make fewer demands so as not to interfere with group feelings and activities.

> I get very emotional, not in the immediate family, in the whole family. If we have any kind of function where it involves the whole family, you're forgotten. 'She can't do this, she can't do that', whereas I can still do lots of things. But no, they just shove me at the back and get on with it, and it hurts not being part of it.
>
> Bobby

Helen often wants other people in her family to make less fuss about her diabetes:

Sometimes with my mother, if I don't feel very well and realize that I need something to eat, I'll go to lengths to disguise it; I'll go to the loo to eat some glucose tablets or say, 'Shall we go and have a coffee?' I'm sure she knows what's going on, but it's like, 'Treat me as normal and I'll be alright', to avoid the fuss or emotional stuff.

Although she is very used to coping with diabetes, Helen has begun recently to see her partner's point of view more and to accept that other people worry because they care:

When we were first together he would overreact and, therefore, I would stop asking for help. We had a situation where I fell down the stairs and ended up with a damaged back because I didn't want to make a fuss! Eventually we sat down and I said, 'All I want is a glass of Lucozade and I'll be perfectly alright. There's no need for any great follow-through.' But on my part, there was the need to explain that rather than to assume that he would know. He said, 'Sometimes you've got to realize that you are a responsibility. You're not being a nuisance or specially different, but someone cares about your well-being and there's a need to respect that.'

Janet also feels that she has a responsibility to others as well as to herself to try and stay as well as possible, because if she is ill, 'Not only does it put a spanner in the works for things I want to do, but it puts a spanner in everybody else's life, who's trying to help me.'

We all struggle with the balance between dependence and independence. Some of us get more from our families than we want and others get less. Marlene talks about what it is like to manage alone:

I've always had to manage since my parents died when I was 14. I stayed with an aunt until I was 16 and then I left. I was virtually on my own for years and years, so I've always been reliant on myself. Even when I was married my husband was often away with his job, so that I couldn't rely on him being around and helping me. I would love to have had somebody as a backstop, somebody looking out for me the way I look out for myself, but I've never had that. It makes me stronger in a way, but it would be nice to be able to relax now and then.

༄

## 'Advised not to have children': starting a family

Finally we come to motherhood and children, the area in which our womanhood is judged and measured more than any other. If disabled women are not supposed to have sex, then it follows that we cannot have children.[3] At a conference on pregnancy, parenthood and disability (organized by the Maternity Alliance), Alison John, a mother of two children who has cerebral palsy, described other people's reactions to her being a mother. At one council meeting a woman said to her, 'Isn't it lovely that you and your husband can adopt children?' to which Alison replied, 'Excuse me, actually we bonked for them' – causing the woman's jaw to hit the floor! Clearly this woman felt that people with cerebral palsy did not have sex, and especially not sex that might result in pregnancy and babies.[4]

Disabled women (in particular women with learning difficulties) may find themselves at risk of sterilization against their will or being prescribed the types of contraceptive which give them least control over their own fertility (such as Depo Provera, the injectable contraceptive).[5] Parents are supposed to be strong, independent and able to care for and protect their children. If disabled women are seen as childlike, dependent and unable to look after themselves, then they will not be seen as fit parents or carers of others. At the same conference, Micheline Mason talked about growing up without any idea that she might leave home and become independent, let alone be responsible for looking after someone else: 'I didn't have the confidence to think I could keep a pot plant alive!' She dedicated her talk to all the disabled people who never made it to parenthood:

> Becoming a parent is the best thing that ever happened to me. I still feel ... that I snatched at something I didn't have a right to.[6]

Of the women I interviewed 11 have children and 16 do not, out of whom perhaps 6 assume they may have them in future, although there might be difficulties. A few women are not unhappy about having no children – one describes herself as 'not kiddy-minded' and another had an abortion as she was adamant that she didn't want children. Most of the women with children had them before they became ill or before their illness was diagnosed; two women have a combination of adopted children and biological children. For some their physical state makes children out of the question, and others have been advised at various times not to have them.

A Maternity Alliance survey reported a number of women who have the same conditions as women in this book (such as rheumatoid arthritis or MS) being told not to have children.[7] It is hard to get accurate information about the impact of pregnancy on various conditions, so that some of us may be unnecessarily frightened of pregnancy and others may not know enough about what the genuine risks are. In this area, as in so many others, medical advice quite reasonably changes over time. Less reasonably, however, advice can vary enormously from one doctor to another; and the potential for doctors to take over control of pregnancy and labour is also greatly enhanced if we are regarded as 'high risk' mothers.

> The first time I was pregnant I went to a specialist. I'd had an attack and I was falling about all over the place. He

wanted to terminate. One didn't do that normally in those days, so I went to another specialist and he said not to terminate but to have a Caesarean. I said, 'Well, that limits my family', and he said I could have four – so I had four.
*Angela*

I was advised not to have children. They wouldn't sterilise me because they didn't know if I would heal, and they couldn't put me on the Pill, so my husband had a vasectomy. Now they know more about the condition, but this is going back 18 years. I did mind because I adore children. I count it as a privilege that we fostered two children for several years.
*Janet*

I had a termination on the advice of a doctor. It was very unpleasant – the staff were insensitive and ill-informed.

The doctor said I would die of AIDS and so would the baby.
*Women with HIV*[8]

For some of us the barriers to having children have been more complex:

When I was a teenager I had a baby and he was adopted, and after I had him I had puerperal psychosis[9]. I had electric shock treatment and was put in a mental hospital, and it did make me very frightened to have a baby again. After I came out of hospital I had what I think were early symptoms of the illness I have now, so I wonder if the psychosis was caused by it as well. In the end I didn't get married until I was 40, and my husband was happy about not having children.
*Shrilly*

Because we were adopting our daughter, I deliberately hid the fact that I was feeling ill and didn't go back to the doctor about things that were concerning me. I was frightened to death that they might say I wasn't fit and it would affect our chances of adopting her, or at the beginning, of adopting at all.

*Patricia*

There is more acceptance these days of women with some kinds of illnesses having children, but only on condition of using all the medical technology available, both to treat us while we are pregnant, and to screen our foetuses for possible defects (so that they don't have to be born). Some of us would like to have children, but are quite frightened about the risks of pregnancy and the practical difficulty of caring for a child when we are ill. Disabled women have justifiable fears about losing their children to the care system:

> I'm not going to have kids until I'm at least 25, because I want to get my health sorted out. I don't want to have fits all the time and not be able to cope and have my child taken off me. What annoys me is that they're quick to take the kids of people who've got illnesses into care, yet there's people who've got nowt wrong with them and their kids are being neglected and badly treated.
>
> *Maureen*

Participants at a conference for women with diabetes wrote afterwards about pregnancy:

> All of us had suffered great fear about pregnancy and childbirth and unanimously agreed there is far too much negative and outdated advice. We are expected to have reached a certain standard of diabetic control in order to have permission to stop using contraception. So we fear having babies with disabilities which will be our fault. We also have immense fears for our own health. Yet among the group all the children were completely healthy and the mothers had no regrets.[10]

## Not a Real Woman?

Grace would like a child, but is not very optimistic about being able to cope without a partner:

> I'd have to be in a more stable physical state and living situation, and have more support around before I could consider it. I'm getting to the age now where the Health Service would call me an elderly primigravida and I would be scarified about my child being disabled and be coerced into having all sorts of tests that I didn't want. The whole prospect is not alluring. The good news is I've got a very lovely cat and I think that's the way it's going to stay!
>
> I think my ambition is just to have some children with someone and be happy. Even if I only had the one child I'll have contributed to the human race. But if I was to marry somebody with sickle-cell anaemia, I wouldn't have them, because I know how much pain I go through every time I have a crisis. It would be OK if I was to have children with the partner I'm with now, because they would just be carriers, they wouldn't have the disease.
>
> *Paris*

> I've always thought that even if I didn't have a partner, by the time I was in my mid-to-late 30s, I would choose to have a child. I would have liked that, but obviously after cancer I couldn't even adopt. I remember a woman in hospital, who had radiotherapy at the same time as me, saying she was sorry for me because I couldn't have any children now. It came as a shock; it had all happened so quickly and nobody had said anything about it. Many women chose radiotherapy rather than surgery because they thought, wrongly, that it would mean children were still possible.
>
> *Lesley*

Maggie's thyroid condition started after she gave birth to her son and was probably triggered by pregnancy. She is frightened of what might happen during another pregnancy. She has had two miscarriages since then and doesn't know whether or not these are connected to her illness. Developing an illness at the same time as having a new baby was also difficult:

> I remember my little boy lying on the carpet and I didn't have the energy to pick him up. It felt that having a new baby was such an enormous thing that being ill as well was a burden I couldn't possibly cope with. I was terror-stricken that I wouldn't be able to cope and that they were going to take my baby away. People expect you to act in a very grown-up way because you're a mother, and it was hard having to remember all the time that I had a much smaller life to look after. It made me really miss my mother, because if she had been alive she would have stepped in and looked after me.

## 'Not what you had kids for': bringing up children

If we do have children, illness is also likely to affect our relationship with them. They may well become more independent or have to help in the house more than other children of the same age. Some of us felt very unhappy about this change in roles:

> I hate it when you see sympathy in their eyes. I don't want to take it away from them about helping out practically, but if I could take away them feeling sorry for me ... I've become somebody to look after and that straight adult/child relationship has gone. I don't like that – it's not what you had kids for. I wish I could drive to this and

that place and do what it seems like every other parent can do with their child. They rely on their dad to do things with them. You don't feel you're 100 per cent a parent.

*Harriet*

When my children were young they were more supportive than my husband was. They would dress me; it would be them I would depend on. My daughter especially was excellent (she is two years older than my son), she was there nearly all the time for me. I didn't realize to what extent my not being able to be there for them was restricting them.

*Mary*

Not all of us, however, saw it as negative that our children helped more with practical things than others did:

> I suppose my sons started learning to do things in their teens, odd bits of shopping, preparing food. The mothers of my younger son's friends thought it was dreadful that I asked him to go to the shops for me, but I think I would have asked him to do things anyway. They're both very good cooks now. They're just the caring types. I think in a way it's been good for them.
>
> *Rachel*

> When people saw me getting into the car and my foster daughter folding up the wheelchair, they would tell me off for being a cruel parent and making her do such awful things for me. But she would say: 'She's not cruel; I enjoy doing it.' She was quite rude, but I thought 'Well, good on you kid!' I find children very capable, very adaptable. One time a disability officer came round, who didn't know that we'd fostered the twins (they were eight years old then), and she remarked: 'No one in their right mind would leave you alone with children' (which I found very hurtful). She

was completely shell-shocked when the twins walked in from school.

*Janet*

Sometimes the main problems experienced by women looking after children were more to do with access to buildings and other people's attitudes than their own energy levels:

My foster son was very much aware of the fact that I couldn't get into the school and went to the headmaster one year to tell him that he wanted me to come to the school play. He just thought they could make it accessible tomorrow! The children were very annoyed that I couldn't get round the school, and I don't think that was fair on them.

*Janet*

There's lots I used to do at the school that I can't do anymore because there's not disabled access. We were quite involved with the older two girls and I find that I'm missing out now with the younger two.

*Bobby*

Bobby and Kabita, who both have diabetes, find that it is difficult combining their own needs and that of the rest of the family, particularly their children:

With the girls at the age they are, with after school activity and homework, meals are staggered and I find it very draining and difficult to cope with. Sometimes I forget to inject because I'm buzzing about doing the meal, and I get really cross that they don't remind me.

*Bobby*

Sometimes I think it makes me scared and sort of impose on the kids, saying 'Look I have diabetes so you've got to be careful what you eat, you should watch your weight', which might not be good for them. When I was diagnosed it took me a long time to come to terms with it, and I was really irritable with the kids and family. There are times when I expect my family to treat me specially because I've got diabetes, which they don't, and I get upset about that.

*Kabita*

Our illness may also create barriers in our physical relationship with children, or as in Joyce's case, grandchildren:

> My grandson loves to be close to me and sit in my lap and hug me, and I feel crowded. He's just showing his love to you but you want to say, 'Sit down, man, and leave me alone.' You just want to sit and be on your own. It pains you in lots of ways.
>
> The kids don't sit on my knee. The cat doesn't sit on my knee, because the weight would kill me!
>
> *Harriet*

Sandra feels very guilty that a combination of mental and physical health problems have prevented her from being as active a parent as she would have liked. She adds, however, that her children are also a reason for getting better: 'I've got my kids to live for, as well as myself to do it for.' This important thought was echoed by Mary, who said that the children are one of the things that have kept her going at times when she has felt most depressed about her illness:

> Pain can bring you very low and there were one or two occasions when I did consider, 'Well, there's no more point in living through it.' But something comes forth, like the children especially, and you get through it.

## 'I know he loves me': positive relationships

Living with illness and living with other people both involve contradictions. We may feel weighed down at times by our sense of dependency and guilt, but along with that comes the security of being loved and cared for. If we have understanding partners, they are probably our greatest source of confidence and support. They are the people we can ask to help us fight battles with doctors or the benefits system. They are the people whose love gives us back our self-esteem when others' attitudes or our own fears take it away:

> Being in a relationship makes me happy. I used to say to my sister that I couldn't get a boyfriend because of the way I walk or because of my illness. She would say, 'Don't be silly, it's because you haven't met the right person yet.' And now I can look back and say, 'Yes, she was right.'
>
> *Paris*

> My current partner is great. He's done a lot for my confidence. When I was on the new insulins, which didn't work for me, at three o'clock in the morning I'd be waving my arms about saying he was trying to kill me while he was trying to get Lucozade down me. And his attitude was: 'What are we going to do about it?', not 'What are *you* going to do?'
>
> *Helen*

> I think between us the relationship hasn't changed. We've just gone on the same way and the relationship has deepened over the years. But I do feel I'm not a partner to him like I was when we first met. We should be doing a lot more things together and enjoying each other a lot more. So I'm always surprised that he likes

me. It's daft. He brought me a bunch of flowers the other day and I thought, 'This guy likes me, still!' When you can't see anything in yourself you're surprised that other people can see something in you.

*Harriet*

The only thing in life that I'm confident about is that I know he loves me, because who would put up with me if they didn't?

*Patricia*

# ~ 5 ~

# *Biting the Hand that Feeds Us: Dealing with the Doctors*

I had four cervical smears during that year but they didn't pick up anything. By the November I was in pain and constantly bleeding, but my doctor wouldn't take any notice. Eventually I saw a gynaecologist who found a stage three carcinoma (which is a very large tumour). He told me and my parents that I was going to die.

*Lesley*

Lesley was then sent for radiotherapy, which was given by a method that was still experimental at the time. The radiotherapy succeeded in destroying the tumour in her cervix but, as for a number of other women, left her with extremely severe internal injuries. The hospital responsible say that the women they treated are lucky to be alive, since they would otherwise have died from their cancer. Lesley can accept this to some extent in her case, since her tumour was very large by the time she was treated, but she disputes it in the cases of many other women. With tumours at an earlier stage, a different form of radiotherapy or a hysterectomy might have offered a chance of survival without such horrific side effects.

Before I was given radiotherapy, I cross-examined the consultant oncologist for about an hour, asking if there were any alternative treatments or any side effects, and he said no. And I really totally believed him. It was my

> life in their hands. Looking back I feel so naive. I was only told the radiotherapy would give me sickness and diarrhoea.

She later found out that they'd introduced a method which had only been tested on mice, and that they were part of a clinical trial without being told; they were experimenting with the doses and method of delivery. After her radiotherapy she asked to see her medical history notes, news of which reached the sister:

> All of a sudden the consultant radiotherapist came to my bedside, held my hand and said, 'I believe you want to see your notes. Don't you trust me?' I said that I was just interested to see them, and he said, 'Honestly, we've given you the best possible treatment.' I was still innocent then so I let him go. But nobody questioned that guy. The nurses thought he was God.

Lesley is one of several women who have started campaigning to get compensation for women who were injured through radiotherapy. Their group, RAGE (Radiotherapy Action Group Exposure) also offers mutual support and raises awareness of the issues. Like other women, Lesley has had many operations to try and repair the damage to her bowel and other internal organs, and has received much good treatment from the same hospital which gave her the radiotherapy. She did not initially want to complain publicly about them, but felt that women's lives were at risk if she and others kept silent:

> I watched a girl in the room next to me die of severe radiotherapy reactions, but I didn't understand then what was going on. When I went in for my main surgery there were three others with me, all in for surgery after radiotherapy, and they're all dead now. We took action in the end because my friend should never have died. She spent her last six months in hospital and I watched

her just go to nothing. She'd had a low-stage tumour, had requested a hysterectomy and been refused. If she'd been given it, she'd probably be alive today. The trauma of diagnosis of cancer is just terrible in itself, but then to find out that the cure has damaged you as well and can kill you ...

This is an extreme example of what can happen to us in the hands of the medical profession. It does illustrate, however, problems that confront many women experiencing serious illness. Screening and other preventive health measures are not infallible: any of us may become ill. Doctors frequently dismiss women patients as neurotic or attention-seeking, even to the extent, as in Lesley's case, of failing to investigate serious and obvious physical symptoms.

Despite continuing developments in medical knowledge and technology, there are rarely easy solutions to serious illness. Treatment often has effects other than those intended: the cure can kill you. It is crucial that we know what we are consenting to, yet the desire to advance medical knowledge may take precedence over the needs or rights of individual patients, and information is often hard to come by. The organization of medical care under different, sometimes competing specialist areas, may militate against us getting the best, most informed treatment. In Lesley's hospital neither the radiotherapists nor the bowel and bladder specialists knew the full possible extent of radiotherapy damage until it began to happen. Even then, however, they apparently were unable to cooperate with one another to work out how best to help the women concerned.

Finally, while cases like Lesley's are certainly not the norm, they do form the backdrop to our experience of health care. Doctors have the power not only of life but also of death over us. It is surely only common sense to fear entrusting ourselves to their care.

## 'My life in their hands': inequality and dependency

If we have a long-term illness, we almost by definition have a long-term relationship with the medical profession. Some of us will have spent much time in hospital, as children and adults. Others may simply see a GP or specialist clinic every so often for tests, prescriptions or sick notes. Some may be able to manage without treatment, or with forms of treatment other than conventional medicine, for long periods of time, before occasionally being thrown back on conventional health care at times of crisis. For nearly all of us, however, the relationship is a part of our lives, a relationship from which we cannot completely escape. We are dependent on doctors for operations and drugs which keep us alive, minimize our symptoms, or control our pain. We also need them to give us official recognition as sick people, to allow us to claim benefits, get appropriate help or equipment, or take time off work.

It is hardly a new observation that the doctor/patient relationship is one fraught with problems, bitterness and resentment on both sides. Indeed many women contributing to this book expressed strong, mostly negative feelings about it:

> Don't talk to me about doctors!
> 
> *Bobby*

> I don't like doctors.
> 
> *Adele*

> Doctors – I just laugh in their faces.
> 
> *Marlene*

Recent decades have seen much work and debate on the way in which women patients are treated in the Health Service.[1]

Like most people in positions of power, most doctors are still male, white and middle class, and often lack the skill or motivation to communicate with and learn from people who are different from them – that is, those of us who are female, black or working class. The medical focus on controlling women's reproductive function is intensified in relation to working class, black and disabled women. Eugenist views and the history of contraception – developed in wealthy countries to limit the reproduction of working-class people at home and black people abroad – have informed medical opinions of the health needs of these groups of women.[2] Medical views about food and weight are also still riddled with prejudice about women and working-class people. There has been positive change, however, and many of us are now more aware of the issue of consent and are better informed about our health, conventional medical treatments and the alternatives. Nevertheless, our ability to get information and assert ourselves in our encounters with doctors still depends heavily on our position in society and level of education, so that much of what has been gained is still out of reach for some women.

Despite these problems, women in this book also have positive experiences and thoughtful analysis to offer of the way in which health care works, arising from our long-term and intimate contact with it. As I mentioned in Chapter 2, women have more frequent and routine contact with the Health Service than men, and for those of us with any kind of chronic or incurable condition, health care is a basic, permanent, routine necessity. We are, therefore, well-placed to comment on both the best and the worst of it.

Women living with long-term illness can obviously claim particular expertise regarding our own health and our own bodies. Each day brings a series of decisions to be made about medication, food, rest or activity. We learn, over many years, perhaps our whole lifetime, how to interpret and manage our body and illness.

> No, they [doctors] are not involved in day-to-day

decisions. You do that yourself. It's just trial and error. You know when you've made a mistake.

*Sade*

You just have to balance it yourself. When you find something that suits you, you stick to it like glue. My biggest urge is please, doctors and nurses, listen to us. Just as a mother knows, nine times out of ten, if there's something wrong with her child, so people with disabilities know when they're suffering and know what helps it.

*Janet*

Yet we are not treated as experienced and equal partners in our own care. We are treated as ignorant of medicine, spoken to as though we were children, threatened with punishment if we do not do as we are told. And like children with their parents, it is hard to fight back because we need these doctors. It simply cannot be overstated how dependent we feel on the various health professionals we deal with and how fundamentally unequal our relationship with them is – a relationship rooted in the difference between strength and weakness:

The GP's very sympathetic, but she's a very active, fit woman, as her job demands, and so there's a gulf between you. You're sat there chronically ill and she's a fit, healthy woman with a full-time job and a million other things to do. In the end you're different.

*Harriet*

It's them and us and I find that quite difficult.

*Bobby*

Of course doctors are only human and do get ill themselves, but this does not fundamentally affect their relationship with us. In fact medical training discourages doctors from identifying with patients. Doctors are supposed to be powerful in combating illness and disease. Illness is equated with weakness and so there is an inherent contradiction in the fact of a doctor being ill. Although we may these days be called 'clients' or 'consumers' rather than the old-fashioned 'patients' (originally meaning 'people who passively suffer'), the reality remains that as ill people we both see ourselves, and are seen by others, as weak and dependent. We can therefore have little or no power in our relationship with those who by definition, by virtue of their power to cure, are strong. We do not have choices, or at least only very limited ones, as to whether or not we use health care, and of course in some ways we are weak because of our illness. We have more limited energy for fighting, for asserting what we want, for looking for the best treatment and care, than we would have if we were well.

> I'm at the stage of saying, 'Well, I've got to find some way of taking responsibility for this myself.' I think it is more difficult now, however, having already had that close contact with the Health Service, because it is so disempowering and undermining. They are so dismissive of any alternative treatment and they scare you about it. So I need to feel well enough to undertake a whole new set of treatments, through diet and exercise, which I'm researching at the moment. But it's the hardest thing, finding the energy to do that when you're ill!
> *Grace*

However, is it not simply a question of our lack of strength. An important barrier to complaining about our treatment or asserting our wishes is that we feel not only dependent, but grateful. Much of the time our experience of health care is one of being cared for. We may have spent much time as an inpatient and outpatient in a particular hospital and have relationships with staff going back for years. They will have looked after us at some of the worst and most vulnerable periods of our lives, and we remember with intense gratitude the things they have done for us:

Hospital's been like a second home to me; marvellous care! Even today with all the shortages you wouldn't know from the nurses or doctors the pressures they're working under. You just get the care, marvellous care.
*Rachel*

The Health Service as a whole has been a bit hit and miss. A couple of times I've been given the wrong blood, as in it's not been my blood type down to a 'T'. Well, I've got very ill with it and obviously if I'd died my mum and dad would have had a case, but because I see them [the Health Service] as looking after me, I don't complain.
*Paris*

Similarly, despite everything that happened to Lesley, it was still a hard decision for her and other women to become involved in campaigning about radiotherapy injuries:

I took part in a video about informed consent and I felt that I was biting the hand that fed me. I felt guilty because the hospital did a lot of brilliant work. But we had no choice but to tell the truth of what had happened, because it had been going on for 15 years and no one had spoken out. Some women didn't even want to know it was the radiotherapy; they were happy not knowing the truth and we kept our mouths shut, we were part of the conspiracy for a long time. We were all frightened that the hospital would be funny with us – you feel so vulnerable in a hospital bed, in your nightie and dressing gown or when you're going into theatre for surgery.

The complaints system in the Health Service in Britain is also not easy to understand, and the odds are stacked against the patient. In some cases of abuse or negligence, a formal complaint and perhaps legal action are clearly necessary. Often, however, what people want is an apology, an assurance that someone coming after them won't face the same problem, or perhaps just access to alternative treatment or a different doctor. The natural tendency of the medical profession to be defensive, secretive and never to admit to a fault militates against such solutions. In addition, the increasing reliance on bringing actions for compensation may also not produce what we most need or want.

> My GP tried to lock me up in the hospital psychiatric unit, because I called her out when I was in severe pain from an arthritis flare up. I made a complaint about her to the British Medical Association, but they said, 'Well, she did refer you to hospital, so we can't do anything.' I wasn't even allowed to be at the hearing.
>
> *Adele*

> I tried to sue my GP for negligence but I backed down from going to the tribunal in the end. This was totally wrong, looking back, but I was frightened. There is a problem as well with medical negligence. It seems that everybody is making money out of it except you. People are being paid vast sums of money for a specialist report, and solicitors are being paid vast sums to do your case for you, and if you end up with nothing at the end, they'll still survive. I believe, ideally, there should be no fault compensation because doctors wouldn't have to be so much on the defensive. If only they could say they were sorry!
>
> *Lesley*

Sade echoes this last point, when speaking of recent problems with doctors and nurses: 'No one ever said they were sorry for doubting my pain. I only wish they could feel it!'

## 'I don't like doctors': limitations of medical care

As a result of experiences like these, and because dealing with the Health Service uses up precious emotional and physical energy, some of us try as far as possible to do without it and to stay away for long periods of time. We may, paradoxically, only go when we are feeling strong, or use it only for very specific purposes, rather than as a general source of support.

> Basically the reason I go to the hospital at the moment is so that somebody's going to say yes, you can have a driving licence and yes, you can have some insurance. And that doesn't actually benefit anybody. If you go to a diabetic clinic there are one or two kids, pregnant women and elderly people. Where are all the others like me? Why do I keep turning up when obviously most people between 20 and 60 don't bother?
>
> *Helen*

> After I developed diabetes I also developed serious compulsive eating. The clinic were no help and just gave me diet sheets. So I stayed away for a couple of years and only went back after the crisis was over, when I'd got my eating under control and lost some weight.
>
> *Woman at a diabetes support group*

It may be that we are able to develop ways of maintaining our health without needing to use the Health Service for drug treatment or surgery. Marlene and Grace have both managed for years at a time to control their rheumatoid arthritis through diet and complementary therapies. Indeed Marlene feels she could have done much more with these if only the necessary information had been made available to her from the start.

Ideally I would like never to have anything to do with them. I've had very good operations, but if I'd known about how I could have improved my health years ago, then I never would have got into that state. I only keep it up because it's terrible to be labelled a difficult patient – if you've turned your back on them, it's your own fault. I've got to be kept on their books in case I ever need to have another operation.

Complementary therapies and diet treatments, however, do not work for everyone and are also too expensive for many of us. For those of us whose impairment is a serious illness, doing without doctors completely is also not usually an option and, from a practical point of view, we may at least want to be 'kept on their books' in case of developments we can't manage ourselves. Changes in the Health Service may make this seem more important than in previous years, as we may worry about being able to get treatment in the future.

Many disabled people who have experienced years of surgery in childhood feel very strongly that the medical profession creates as many problems as it cures, perhaps sometimes more. The history of women's health care is also littered with debates about the validity of various operations and procedures, especially those performed on female organs, such as hysterectomies and mastectomies, of which surgeons seem so fond, and especially those apparently done for preventive rather than curative purposes. There is nowadays increasing publicity about the phenomenon of iatrogenesis – that is, illness or injury caused by medical treatment, and a continual supply of horror stories about medical maltreatment in the media. Small wonder if many of us approach hospitals or clinics with fear and loathing!

I had a run-in with a consultant who was about to do a biopsy for lung cancer. My GP had said the right lung, so when I saw him going for my left side with the needle I said, 'Hang on a minute!' He stormed out in a huff and it turned out it was the left lung, but I said, 'There's no need to treat me like the village idiot. I was told the right side.' After all, they have been known to amputate the wrong limb, haven't they?

*Woman at a cancer support group*

Besides all this, and however little we think that doctors know or care, that fact remains that they are probably the people most closely involved with our illness apart from ourselves. We have knowledge based on experience and they have medical knowledge of our disease. Few other people around us will know much, unless we are in a self-help or support organization. Our angry, fighting talk and dismissive remarks are only part of the picture. While we remain tied into the relationship we continue to need things from it, both practically and emotionally. If our doctor is the only other person who can be expected to take an interest in our cancer, diabetes or arthritis, then our feelings of grief and rage if they are dismissive or judgmental will be all the more intense. We may not always like them, but we may want and need their approval and support. One of the strongest themes emerging from women's accounts of their dealings with doctors is that of being cast off or left alone to deal with our illness in isolation.

No one said a word to me [after a mastectomy] except 'Come back in three weeks' time.' It was only when I saw the district nurse that she said I should be getting pain relief. I couldn't move my arm at all. My husband's not even been in St John's Ambulance, but he worked out exercises for me, and I got my arm up. I think that was wrong. I think we should have been given some help in that direction, not have had to do it ourselves.

*Woman at cancer support group*

The doctors weren't sympathetic, they just couldn't understand what I was trying to tell them. In the early days I did feel very alone and very isolated.

*Maggie*

> One doctor I didn't like at all. She was very ignorant. She's only nice to the women that are having babies, that's all. Anyone else, she just treats them like there's nothing wrong with them. When I went to her because I was applying for disability living allowance she just said, 'Oh, you don't need this. You're a lot fitter than that.' Her attitude just stank. I was also in hospital a couple of months ago having tests to see why I keep having fits, why they're not controlled, but they haven't told me anything. They're still not controlled. I'm on these tablets but they're doing no good.
>
> *Maureen*

So Maureen has been left feeling that first her need for basic income, and now her health needs, have been ignored by the people who are supposed to help her. Several of us talked about doctors 'liking' some sorts of patients and not others, and very few of us think we are the sort they like. We are too assertive, too unique, too ordinary, too time-consuming, too neurotic, the wrong class, or in some other way just not what we feel the doctor is interested in:

> Unless I can present myself as really interesting or exciting, or having something particularly wrong at any one time, well, I'm just another diabetic.
>
> *Helen*

Some of us have felt particularly let down by doctors' apparently brusque and dismissive attitudes at the time of our diagnosis:

> He just told me I was going to die.
>
> *Woman at a cancer support group*

> He was alarmist and told me, 'Don't have children, don't be in a car crash.' He treated me like a leper; he didn't give hope and comfort, just doom and gloom.
>
> *Woman with HIV*[3]

And they said, 'You have spina bifida occulta, a severe form of sciatica. You are never going to work again, you will be in a wheelchair by the age of 25 (I was just coming up to 21 at this time). There is a possibility of damage to the legs which could need amputation or further operations, but we can't help you. So you can come back if you want, but really it's a waste of our time and yours.'

*Adele*

One of the most difficult situations for doctors to deal with is a problem which they cannot cure. Modern Western medicine is based on a curative model, and often seems unclear about its role in relation to long-term incurable illness, unhappy when confronted with its limitations. While we may feel that as patients we still need or want contact with the medical profession, they may not want this contact, as in Adele's case, perhaps because it reminds them that they are not all-powerful. Eleanor found herself a rarity when she suffered a very severe stroke at the age of 25, but recovered sufficiently to want to go back to work:

At every stage I'm so unusual they don't know what will happen, what effects all the drugs will have, whether I'll have another stroke and so on. I'm untreatable and so nobody wants to know. Doctors like patients where they can be little gods and say, 'You've got such and such and I can do this for you and then you'll be alright.' I'm too unique to be of interest, the doctor at the pain clinic just said, 'Don't come back because I can't do anything for you.' Now he's being very supportive and helpful. I think it's finally got through to him that I don't expect him to wave a magic wand and that I don't think any the less of him because he can't wave this magic wand.

*Eleanor*

The sense of desertion and rejection may at times be shared by people experiencing acute short-term illness, when they get less information, attention, follow-up and reassurance than they want. However, if an acute illness or injury is resolved and we get better, any negative experiences of health care will become less important over time, and will not be crucial in the long term to our sense of self-worth. For those living with chronic illness, rejection or disapproval by medical professionals is often experienced over and over again, and does reinforce our sense of low worth or importance in the world. As we discussed earlier, observing our own body and the multiple different factors influencing its behaviour is a complex, often tedious and lonely affair, and it is hard to know if we are doing everything right. We need informed, non-judgmental reassurance and support. We need to feel that we are not completely alone with our illness, especially since the very fact of having developed an illness may lead us to worry more about our health and need more reassurance than we might have done when we were well.

> I would like more regular check-ups because you do worry more about your health if you know you've got something wrong with you.
>
> *Maggie*

> With every ache and pain you think, 'Oh my God, cancer again', even if you're getting the flu.
>
> *Woman at a cancer group*

> Because I have all these vague aches and pains, there's a tendency to put everything down to the same thing. I worry that if I had something seriously wrong with me I might not recognize it. Or I might go pestering about something that I feel is serious and it's not. So I'm frightened of them thinking I'm wasting their time and also of missing something serious. Everybody worries about serious illness, but when you feel croaked most of the time, it's difficult to distinguish between what's just a bad

day and what's something else coming. So that I do find very hard.

*Patricia*

## 'He never stopped answering my questions': good experiences of health care

Our dealings with the medical profession are not all negative, however. Some of us have very good experiences of health care and good relationships with doctors and other professionals. In talking of these, the words which come up again and again are: 'partnership', 'trust' and 'listening'. These themes are common in public sector jargon these days but many people regard this as rhetoric rather than indicating a real change in culture. The medical profession would do well to listen harder to what it is that these women mean when they talk about such things. What we want to help us cope with living long term with complicated and often frightening conditions is a sense of partnership: a pooling of information from both sides, a joint attempt to understand and manage a complex situation, and a sense of trust and mutual responsibility for our well-being.

> My GP is wary of saying anything contra the consultant, but she's supportive and will make useful suggestions. That's what I want, that partnership; 'I have a certain amount of information and what can you do to help?'
>
> *Helen*

> My GP and I are now building a good relationship. I know an awful lot about my condition that I've picked up over the years, and he knows that by talking to me he will find out an awful lot more.
>
> *Adele*

So we want doctors to listen to us, to take serious account of the information we have from our own experience of our illness. We also want them to give us information. There is more emphasis these days on patient education at the point of diagnosis, at least with some illnesses or conditions. However, we may need information at different points in our lives. We should be able to ask questions and access information whenever we need to. We also want to be told honestly about side effects of treatments, and not be offered bland reassurances or simply be left in the dark.

> The eye clinic is excellent, brilliant. Even though they have had NHS cuts, I know that I can ring up and they'll say, 'Yes, we'll see you.' They'll spend an awful lot of time explaining what's happening, and will say honestly what's likely to happen in the future.
> *Helen*

> The bowel surgeon is wonderful. I asked loads and loads of questions. He never stopped answering my questions or made me feel silly for asking them.
> *Lesley*

We are very grateful for doctors and nurses who will take the time to listen to our worries and difficulties. Some of us may not need this because we have family and friends to talk to, but we may be on our own, or simply find that people close to us have difficulty in understanding things about our illness. Kabita gets a sense from her doctor that he understands the complexities of her life a little, that he doesn't blame her for not always finding diabetes easy to deal with (or for putting on weight, for instance), and feels that it is precisely because he is not close to her but a doctor with wide experience of the disease that he is able to do this:

> The consultant was really good. He took time to explain. I told him a lot of things about how I felt, things my husband and my closest friend didn't know. He had a

listening ear to talk about it and share it. I think he understands because he sees a lot of patients and there might be some like me. He is good and I also saw the diabetic nurse and she had a lot of information. She gave me the telephone number so that if I was worried about anything I could ring her.

My doctor will listen to me, whatever I want to say. You can sit in his surgery and you feel alright.

*Joyce*

I get great comfort from her, which I've never felt about doctors before. It's just what I need. Not that you want to moan, but you just want someone to flaming well listen. If something happened, I could go to her. She'd be serious with me. She'd know I wasn't putting it on.

*Harriet*

Harriet touches here on the importance of being taken seriously – our need to have our expertise about our own illness recognized and to be treated as responsible adults. This may not seem like much to ask, but those of us who do have a good relationship with our doctor, one based on trust and respect, are acutely aware of how rare this is and how lucky we are:

Yes, I feel in control of my health to a certain degree, but I think that's because I'm very fortunate in having a good GP. He'd prefer me to have a good quality of life and get rid of the pain. I'm on a pain-relieving drug that is addictive, but I cut it down and increase it myself, and he trusts me to do that. I think trust is very important.

*Janet*

Some of what we are talking about is simply down to personality and communication skills, some of it requires fairly major changes in attitude in the medical profession, and some of it is to do with resources and the organization of health care. None of us are demanding many more hours of time overall with our doctors or nurses, but simply the recognition that there may be points of crisis or change when we do need a lot of time. Often all we want is the assurance of knowing that we can get access to advice or treatment quickly and easily if we need it.

> He gave me all the support I needed while I was coming off the antidepressants and then the tranquillizers. If I got in a panic attack, he'd let me call him out, and he gave me a phone line I could phone him on any time that I wanted.
>
> *Sandra*

> The rheumatologist came to my house at 10.30 p.m. one night because I was having quite a few problems. He couldn't sort it out, so the next day he saw me in the day room on the ward while he was doing his rounds. He's quite obliging.
>
> *Mary*

This is written at a time of immense change in the UK Health Service, about which almost every woman I spoke to expressed concerns and fears. However, the more positive changes noted by some of us in recent years concern our relationship with professionals, greater availability of information and people to talk to, and more flexible systems which make access to treatment easier:

> Definitely there's been a great change in attitude. They feel they have to explain things to you and that they can't act like God. And also, of course, I can get my [medical] notes now, if I wanted to.[4]
>
> *Marlene*

> At my doctor's practice there are people there if you want to see them. There is much more information, and they can spread themselves a bit more now that

somebody can go in and talk to a nurse without having to make an appointment with the doctor; it somehow feels better if you're not having to take up the doctor's time. I think that has improved things for a lot of people.

*Patricia*

I've got self-admission now. Usually I self-admit to the ward, whereas before I'd been waiting around in hospitals for hours and hours for pethidine, when I'd been in absolute extreme pain.

*Paris*

Some of our best experiences are in specialist clinics where staff get to know us. Because of the stigma attached to people who are HIV positive, there is a need for clinics where patients can be sure of well-informed staff who will respect confidentiality. Some women in the survey carried out by Positively Women[5] described the benefits of being able to get most of their health needs met in one place. Anna also very much appreciates this service:

> The hospital I go to has a clinic, where they try and make it really nice for you. I can phone up and see my own consultant within a couple of weeks and if something happens I can go straight up there and check it out. If I wanted to see about diet and everything I think I'd get that information, and the hospital now offers appointments with a homoeopath and massage and the like. To see a homoeopath actually working with the doctors, that's not bad! They've got a brilliant nurse there who can see if you're upset and will say, 'Sit down and talk this one out.'

*Anna*

So, what we get from our health care when it is good, is people to listen to us without judging us, a sense of being trusted and having our experience and knowledge respected, and information to make it possible to take realistic and conscious decisions about our own health and treatment. The reason that so little of this chapter deals with positive experiences is that, unfortunately, most of us, most of the time, have not had these experiences. Among all the things we are looking for, getting the information we need and want seems one of the hardest tasks we have to face.

## 'If you don't ask, they don't tell you': the search for information

If they do a blood test they don't tell you what the result is. If you don't ask they don't tell you.

*Tracey*

Many a time I wonder what I really know about this thing? You go and they prescribe tablets for you. They say, 'Don't eat this and don't eat that', but why are you not to eat it? I've never had anybody sit down and say, 'Look, this thing is such and such and is dangerous, and the reason why we said you're not to eat this or that is because this and that will happen.' I feel so ill some days and I'm worried about my eyes. I've been on these tablets so long I don't think they're doing me any good. I don't know what's happening.

*Joyce*

Many of the women speaking in this book have been able to get hold of information to help them understand their illness, but may still feel angry that they have had to work so hard to find it, and that it was not freely available through the Health Service. Others, even after years of living with an illness, still don't have enough information to be able to look after themselves properly. We may be told things that are simply inaccurate, or be told the basics but not in a way that leaves us feeling confident in handling the day-to-day complexities of our condition. It may be that we are given information in language we do not understand, or that doctors assume we cannot understand and so do not bother to explain. We may each need to be told things in different ways.

Doctors are rarely skilled in speaking in simple English. Sade is a nurse, but even she has found it difficult:

> When I was first diagnosed, I couldn't understand what the doctors were saying. It was right over my head, too technical and complicated. Now I know a lot more about it, so I can really question them. And they don't like it, they don't like it at all. They say a bit of knowledge is a dangerous thing, but I think I've a right to know.
>
> As a person you become, over the years, a little different, more forthright, and it's easier to ask. Even now you have to pin them down and say, 'Tell me. I want to know.' They skirt around you and you've to ask quite forthrightly. I want to know everything and I ask questions. I feel awful sorry for people that don't have the forceful personality to push themselves forward. It must be very difficult.
>
> *Mary*

Even when we are quite assertive, as Mary says she has become, getting information out of the medical profession can seem as hard as getting the proverbial blood from a stone. Over and over again in different interviews women said, 'But what about the other women, who can't stand up for themselves, who aren't able to ask questions?' Older women, women who can't speak English well or who don't have a high level of education, women who are just less confident, more frightened of or respectful towards doctors just don't get told things because they don't ask. They are also not treated in a way that encourages them to feel they have the right to ask:

> I'm horrified at the way they speak to older people, the lack of respect shown to these 70-year-old people. You hear somebody yelling at them,' You've been eating!'
>
> *Helen*

So women may go to outpatient appointments every few months, have blood tests but not be told the results and leave none the wiser about what is happening to them. They don't like to ask questions or voice worries because they know the consultant is busy and he (or occasionally she) doesn't offer information. Community health workers such as district nurses, dieticians or physiotherapists who visit people in their homes, may fill in some of these gaps in information. As a system, however, this is frighteningly patchy and dependent on individuals' knowledge and communication skills. In addition, financial cuts and reorganization in health care have undermined community health services:

> I used to have a community physiotherapist coming to see me, then an occupational therapist and a social worker. It felt like a sort of network and I got information that way. Now, if I don't keep up with things myself, nobody will look out for me.
>
> *Marlene*

A different problem is that they may not have the information we want, perhaps because medicine simply doesn't know the answers yet, because our illness is rare or only recently discovered, or because each individual will respond to a disease differently.

> I've got cancer in my spine and I wear a corset most of the time. I want to get some time without the corset, but I daren't do much without the consultants – but I don't think they know either because everybody's individual. If

I did without it, after I've cooked tea and washed up, I might jolt or jerk – would I be paralysed again? I don't think they know.

> *Woman at a cancer support group*

I think I give my surgery more information on lupus than they've ever given me.

> *Shirley*

They don't know anything that I want to know about arthritis (like what causes it), so what can they talk about? It's like taking your car to a garage where they don't know anything about the make of car you drive!

> *Marlene*

HIV is an obvious example of a disease that is fairly new and about which the medical profession, and people who are HIV positive themselves, still have much to learn. Women with HIV or AIDS will also find their care affected not only by ignorance but also by immense prejudice among health workers. As Anna points out, if the Health Service is still so uninformed about it, is it any wonder that the general public doesn't understand it well?

> It was pretty awful getting diagnosed with HIV back then (nine years ago). I had one good doctor and he was fine, and one good interview with a health worker who was brilliant and knew her stuff. But all the rest were absolutely useless. My worry is that if I become ill and have to go into hospital, I may end up in one where they don't have specialist wards. I don't want to end up on any old ward, tagged in a corner. There's still a huge amount of ignorance among health staff around HIV.

Anna's fears are borne out by the experience of women interviewed by Positively Women:

> The hospital orderlies wouldn't come into my room. People were scared to use the same cups, knives etc. There was general ignorance and fear.[6]

Those with AIDS are not the only ones who come up against ignorance and prejudice. Sickle-cell anaemia is an inherited blood disease almost exclusively affecting black people. This means that in parts of the UK with small black populations, health professionals may have little or no experience of it, and racist attitudes may influence how people with sickle-cell anaemia are treated in hospital. Campaigning by the black community has helped to raise awareness of the disease and, over the years, Paris has noticed improvements in how well-informed health workers are:

> They make mistakes because they don't know enough about the condition, and it's difficult because I'm probably the only sickler in the area. Mostly they know that I know more about it – I always carry a book about sickle cell and sometimes the nurses ask if they can look at it. But they are more informed than they used to be. Before, if one of us went into hospital asking for something for the pain, people would look at you as if you were a junkie. Now they know that it's genuine pain, that you're not faking it and that you need the painkillers. Up until last year the nurses always used to say, 'Again?!' when I asked for more pain relief.

Janet has a rare connective tissue disorder (EDS) and is used to meeting ignorance among health workers. Like Paris, she often finds herself in situations where she knows more about EDS than the people treating her, which can be a frightening degree of responsibility to have when you are ill:

> If I go into hospital for anything, nine times out of ten I come out worse than I went in because of the lack of education [about EDS]. So I try to avoid them as much as I can. Recently I had to go to a casualty department

and the doctor had heard of EDS but not come across it, so I showed him the cards that I carry. But he wasn't very cooperative, it didn't help much.

Sometimes this ignorance could be overcome by improved training within the Health Service, but there is also a more fundamental problem – that women's health and illness has generally been of relatively little interest to the medical profession. Men are more frequently the subjects of medical research than women (except of course in the area of reproduction). So information available to doctors themselves may be inadequate or inaccurate because it is based on research done on men, and women's experience is then simply assumed to be the same.[7] Many women with diabetes, for example, find that their blood sugar levels and, therefore, their insulin requirements vary at different points of the menstrual cycle. We have usually had to discover this for ourselves, however, and then worked out how to deal with it:

> I've got a thing about the menstrual cycle, it causes diabetics horrendous problems. I don't know whether consultants don't find that very exciting or whether it's because most of them are men, but it's: 'Well, test your blood a bit more, dear, and you'll be alright.'
>
> *Helen*

The study of AIDS is another example of this problem. The list of symptoms drawn up in the US during the 1980s as indicating HIV and AIDS remained for a long time based on symptoms reported by gay men, the first group known to have the disease. Kaposi's sarcoma is probably the symptom best known to many health workers and to the public, often used to symbolize the stigma of AIDS – yet it is rarely seen in women. Instead infections such as thrush, cystitis or pelvic inflammatory disease are common in HIV-positive women, but have often been treated by health professionals as simply routine gynaecological problems which women get anyway. This may be one reason why women tend to get diagnosed later in the stage of the disease and why women's survival time after diagnosis is shorter than men's.[8]

As I mentioned early on in the book, this problem of a lack of appropriate or relevant information may be magnified for black women, lesbians, disabled women or others who fall outside what is considered the 'normal' group of women. Information may not be available in a language or form we can read, diet advice may not take account of our culture and usual diet. Alternatively, it may simply be that since we don't appear in the literature, it is hard for us to know whether or not it relates to us. Audre Lorde wrote in *The Cancer Journals* of the dearth of information or advice about breast cancer and mastectomy which spoke to her as a black woman and a lesbian.[9] Paula Fenton Thomas has written of her experience of developing lupus as a black woman in Britain. Lupus is an autoimmune disease affecting women more frequently than men and black people more than white. Its symptoms are many and varied, which has caused problems for several women in this book in getting diagnosed.

> When I was told I had lupus ... I was told that it was a rare blood disease 'common to black females in the northern states of America'. I wondered how on earth I had got it ... Six years after my diagnosis, I met many white sufferers of lupus when I went to my first conference on the disease ... There was no reference to black people, except for the presence of one black woman in a slide which was shown ... There was no information about black people in the leaflets that were available.[10]

And finally, many women have complained of the difficulty of getting information on alternative treatments from the Health Service. Marlene's experience is that this information has either not been available or was not offered to her, and Grace has similar frustrations:

> They don't tell you what you can get. You have to know about it and then ask. They say, 'Is there anything you'd

like?' and I say, 'Well, you could send me to the South of France for a month' – which of course they can't – but what I'd really like is if they'd say, 'Well no, we can't do that, but we can let you have acupuncture.' But no, they don't say that. I've only got the course of acupuncture as a result of going to a pain clinic.

*Marlene*

When I asked for advice about diet (because it seemed to me that colitis was something that could well be helped by diet), first of all the view was that it was irrelevant (so I didn't get to see a dietician), then the consultant recommended a diet which was discredited for this condition in the 1950s! In the end, I found a self-help book and talked to women I know with experience of a similar condition.

*Grace*

## 'It's "Rest!" from one doctor and "Exercise!" from another': communication problems

Living with chronic illness involves having to deal with quite complex medical situations. For many of us the treatment we are on causes problems. Drugs to control epilepsy have made Maureen put on weight, for example. Steroids also cause weight gain and raise blood glucose levels, so that it is possible that Bobby's diabetes was caused by long-term steroid use for her asthma. Long-term use of other anti-inflammatory drugs and of various painkillers can cause ulcers or other digestive problems, and many drugs become less effective with constant use or carry the risk of addiction. In addition, as I have already said, no two individuals are completely alike in their response to a particular illness or treatment. So we need accurate, informed and sophisticated medical advice to help us deal with these issues, advice which takes full account of the information we have from our own lived experience.

> The most frightening aspect of the whole experience was when they started me on the treatment; because my thyroid level was so low, it turned out to be much too high a dose of thyroxin for me. Within a few hours I was getting muscle spasms in my legs, pins and needles in my feet, my face was flushing and I thought I was going to have a heart attack. The doctor I saw said there were no side effects of the treatment and that my reaction was psychosomatic. I was extremely upset about this. I felt that it was treated quite lightly, given how ill I was feeling. I thought I was flipping my lid at one point.
> *Maggie*

> It's complicated and a lot of times you don't know why you feel like this. I get anxiety attacks, really bad pains in my chest, where I think I'm going to have a heart attack – but the doctor says there's nothing wrong that he can see.
> *Sandra*

Many of us have felt extremely frustrated at the lack of a holistic approach within health care – that is, an approach that looks at the whole experience of a person, and so can take account of the interaction of different conditions and treatments, as well as the other things going on in our lives and affecting our minds and bodies. A friend recently talked to me about being treated for endometriosis (a long-term gynaecological condition which can cause fertility problems) and receiving in vitro fertilization (IVF) treatment, at the same time and in the same hospital – but with no coordination between the two departments. She had to find out for herself that one of the drugs she was on for endometriosis could in itself cause difficulties in conceiving. Women who have more than one condition clearly have a particularly difficult time managing their health and treatment. The lack of coordination between specialists, together with the attitudes of some doctors, only make the task more difficult. This can prevent us getting complete information, may slow down the process of diagnosis or mean that treatments are conflicting with each other.

> I had ulcer treatments and treatments for my eyes and all the different symptoms, but nobody ever seemed to put it all together – they all seemed to think they were just nothing to do with one another.[11]
>
> *Shirley*

> A lot of women go straight from the district hospital gynaecologist, who's used to the menopause and hysterectomies (and thinks, 'Oh God, I don't want to deal with this'), to a radiotherapist, who is biased about the treatment and won't offer anything but radiotherapy.
>
> *Lesley*

Patients are often blamed for failing to follow medical instructions. Yet how are we supposed to cope with conflicting advice from different specialist consultants and nurses? Janet has multiple sclerosis as well as EDS, and Bobby has diabetes, asthma, rheumatoid arthritis and has had two heart attacks:

> There's conflicting medicines that you can have. The MS is helped by steroids, but they make the connective tissue side of it (the EDS) worse, because steroids break down your skin tissue so you can start having sores again. You have to weigh up very carefully. If I go to hospital they'll just try and put you in a little box and say it's because of the EDS or it's because of the MS and they won't bother to investigate any further. I find that quite frustrating because, nine times out of ten, I know which is the problem.
>
> *Janet*

It's 'Rest!' from one doctor and 'Exercise!' from another – and they're all in the same hospital, you'd think they could talk to each other! I said the other day that I'm not going again unless they sort it out. They shove you your tablets and you say, 'They're going to interrupt my sugar level', and they say, 'Oh no, you'll be alright', not 'Right, we'll sit down and work that out.' You're just left.

*Bobby*

Bobby also had problems with her weight, with doctors on the one hand telling her to lose weight (which she'd do), and then on the other putting her on steroids (which would make her gain weight), without taking this into consideration. When she was admitted to hospital she also found the sister telling her that she did not need special meals, and the dietician saying that she did. In the end, her partner would bring her in sandwiches for tea:

You do as best as you can at home, but you expect that in hospital it'll be there, it'll be done for you. Luckily I'm not a stupid person so we try and work it out, but what about people who panic? They're just given these tablets, just get on with it ... very naughty, I think.

Medical advice and treatment also vary between hospitals and different parts of the country, and fashions come and go in medical belief and advice. Because Helen has had diabetes since the age of five and has lived in several different parts of the UK, she has observed enormous changes over time in how diabetes is treated, as well as differences between one hospital and another, one consultant and another:

It's as though consultants get excited about the new thing and so give out the same advice to all their patients. I wouldn't say I have a respect, but I do have an interest in what consultants have to say, like: 'What's the latest thing on diabetes? What's the latest test?' I can enter into that kind of dialogue with them.

Every hospital gives different radiotherapy to women, even when the cancers are the same.

*Lesley*

It is hard for most people to keep up with and respond to these changes, and we are not particularly helped by inconsistent and sometimes sensationalist reporting in the media. The degree of dogmatism with which doctors give out their advice, even as it changes from one decade to the next, also serves mainly to make people feel disempowered, apathetic and uncertain about what they should be doing. Living through these decades of changing treatment and attitudes to our disease, we may simply become resigned to there being no simple right answer. There is, of course, progress in both medical knowledge and technology, along with improvements in treatment which patients themselves have lobbied for, but good things may get thrown out with the bad, and it can appear as if professional needs and interests come before our own.

The structure and organization of health care also get in the way of women getting what we want. Our awareness of the pressures on doctors discourages us from taking up too much of their time. We may mind less having to wait for long periods in outpatient clinics than the fact we get only a few minutes with the doctor, although the general assumption that our time is less valuable than that of health professionals may be just one of the many ways in which they undermine our self-esteem and sense of being cared for:

It's as quick as they can get me in and get me out. And I hate being treated in that way, it's so degrading. You're just a number or something.

*Mary*

I'd just get him for two minutes and I couldn't explain all these funny symptoms – he'd be rushing out. I don't think it's altogether his fault because he's got about a thousand patients waiting outside.

*Shirley*

Medical hierarchies also get in the way of effective communication between patients and the medical profession. Some of us have developed good relationships with consultants, who are likely to be both the most knowledgeable and the least approachable of the health professionals we encounter. Other women have found junior doctors easier to deal with, 'the small men', as Mary put it, more useful 'than the higher ones, the professors and that'. The profession as a whole, however, certainly includes fine examples of the arrogance both of youth and age. Relationships within the profession are mystifying, unappealing and alienating for us as patients, and seem to have little or nothing to do with our needs and treatment.

> I find junior doctors are willing to understand but the consultants just dismiss what the junior doctors are saying – especially if the consultant's an older person, they seem to think they know it all. They sort of get stuck in their little tracks and go along that line quite happily. They are not going to take a branch line off it or have any other viewpoints at all.
>
> *Janet*

> I was shocked at the extent to which the same hierarchies are there that I used to see in *Carry On Doctor* films. The consultant comes round and all the patients must be sat up in the beds looking alert. It's all flurrying about and kowtowing all over the place, talking about me across the bed, grilling junior doctors about diagnosis.
>
> *Grace*

## 'This patient refuses to relinquish control of her treatment': regaining our power

So how do we deal with this problematic relationship? What ways do we find to maintain or acquire some sense of control over our own bodies? Some women feel that the only sensible course is to deal with doctors as we would be dealt with and be as honest as possible. Honesty can be a risky policy however. We can give information to our doctors but we cannot force them to interpret it correctly. We also have little or no control over the information we give them. For some of us the risks are too great, but others believe that withholding information also carries risks. If we are open with them, then at least we have done our best to improve the relationship.

> I try and honestly say what my problems are and see whether anything comes out of it. A lot of diabetics are not honest with their consultants because of the responses that they get. I think with being working class, and a woman, we're brought up to respect doctors more, and in a certain way diabetes has helped me with assertion – sitting with a doctor across a table and suggesting that they may be wrong, there may be other options, or just that no, I haven't been a naughty girl.
>
> *Helen*

Some of us are either by nature or through bitter experience confrontational and assertive. As already said, those with rare or complicated conditions may well become more knowledgeable than the doctors they see, which in itself may give them the strength and confidence to stand up to doctors. Both Adele and Eleanor know a lot about their conditions, what works and doesn't work for them, and both are prepared, in different ways, to stand up to doctors when they are certain that they are wrong or that they are not getting what they need.

> I challenge them. I will go in, look them straight in the eye and I demand satisfaction. This specialist ordered a lumbar puncture (considered very dangerous for me) without actually asking me. I was prepared to bring in a solicitor over this and it frightened him. I will not brook any nonsense from any doctor. If I'm sat in a hospital bed with a specialist and several hundred students talking about me over my head, I will intervene and very brusquely tell that specialist, 'Speak my language or discuss me out of earshot.' Because patients are intimidated by them, the ones like me come as a bad shock. I don't like doctors. I think they should all be put in a field and bombed.
>
> *Adele*

Eleanor read medical books on her condition which, along with her working experience in hospitals, has armed her with a knowledge of medical terminology and how the system works:

> I try and impress this idea of us being a partnership; it works better if I find out what I can and then suggest to them, 'Perhaps this would work. What do you think?' The doctor I'm registered with now is very nice and doesn't seem to mind me suggesting things. There's no reason why they should really. It's my life and it's my body. One consultant wrote, 'This patient refuses to relinquish control of her treatment', and I said, 'He's dead right I won't!' Why should I just let them do what they want? Looking at my medical history, they've done nothing but make a bigger mess of me.
>
> *Eleanor*

## Biting the Hand that Feeds Us

Direct confrontation or blatant refusal to comply with medical advice may often be taken as a sign of irresponsibility or even mental instability, a label which we know can seriously damage our health. Doctors complain bitterly about patients lying to them, but sometimes an indirect, dishonest, but polite approach seems the best way through the maze.

> I feel more in control now that I know the doctors aren't going to try and give me drugs, because years ago they wanted to. I didn't want to be labelled a difficult patient, so I used to pretend to take them, or else look up the side effects and pretend to have them, so they'd take me off them. Only recently I found out that my notes said they didn't think I was taking the tablets – so I wasn't fooling them altogether. It wasn't that I wanted to make fools out of them, but I didn't want to be in a position where I was forced to take drugs.
>
> *Marlene*

So we find ways to handle our relationship with the medical profession as individuals, but we can also get help from others. One very basic thing that can make a difference is to take a friend or partner with you when you have a hospital appointment which you are worried about. Even if they say nothing, their presence in the consulting room may feel protective – they can act as a witness if nothing else. The power difference between us and the doctor can be subtly altered, and many doctors are much more polite in the presence of a third party.

We have talked of the difficulties of getting information and how some women, like Eleanor or Marlene, have helped themselves by becoming very well informed about their respective conditions. Places such as Well Women clinics or women's health groups may be able to provide information and advice, as can Community Health Councils[12], specialist self-help groups and some medical charities. Besides equalizing the imbalance of knowledge between us and our doctor, the mere fact of having talked to someone informed but outside the Health Service, or the sense of belonging to a group, may make us feel far more confident and able to be assertive (perhaps also even calm and polite!) Community Health Councils and advocacy groups (such as the Patient's Association or Action for Victims of Medical Accidents in the UK) can also offer advice if we find ourselves in the extreme situation of having to make a complaint or take legal action against the Health Service. Most women in this book have, at one time or other, received help or support from friends or from these kind of organizations.[13]

## 'He called me a silly woman and put me on the Pill': denial and disbelief

Another common thread running through women's experiences is that of doctors not believing women when they report worries or symptoms of illness:

> It was such a relief to get a diagnosis. In a way you shouldn't need a name, you should be able to just be ill – but you do need it because otherwise you have to face the attitude that you're just a young silly woman who is depressed. They kept trying to give me antidepressants.
>
> *Clare*

Some of us have had relatively straightforward experiences of diagnosis. We go to our doctor, explain our symptoms, they listen and try to make a diagnosis. However several women have spent years dealing with suspicion and disbelief from doctors. It is maybe so commonplace as not to need saying, that women are not listened to by the medical profession or by society in general. However, the reality of this still has the power to shock when looking at individual women's experiences and the effect that denial and disbelief have had on their health. The moment of getting a diagnosis of an incurable condition, when we face the reality of something which will change our lives forever, can be devastating. However nothing, it seems, is as bad as not knowing and not being believed:

> The consultant was great. It was so easy; she took me seriously. I'd had years and years of doctors saying, 'We don't really know what's wrong with you', saying stupid things like, 'Maybe you're breathing too fast and making yourself faint, try breathing into a plastic bag.' Or they'd ask if things always happened at the same time of the month and I'd think, 'No, you're on the wrong track here, I can see it'll be hot flushes next.' When we got the diagnosis, my doctor said she was sorry she sent me, but I said, 'I'm glad you sent me because now I know I'm not mad.' To me it's important. I've spent so many years thinking, 'Is it me?'
>
> *Harriet*

Our fear of madness is exacerbated by the tendency of the medical profession to put women's complaints of physical symptoms down to mental health problems. A recent study comparing treatment of men and women with heart disease found that women are far more likely to have their initial symptoms dismissed as psychosomatic and, therefore, to be denied appropriate treatment.[14]

> Rheumatic things are vague – not something the doctor can see – so from the start you feel like a neurotic woman who's got nothing better to do with her time than grumble about her health.
>
> *Patricia*

> I know another woman with ME who had electric shock treatment for two months and was kept in psychiatric

care because she was not believed about it being a physical illness.

*Clare*

My doctor's very sympathetic, but even he thought I'd got postnatal depression and would have treated me for that if I hadn't mentioned my mother having an underactive thyroid.

*Maggie*

We may manage to resist antidepressants or more dramatic psychiatric treatment, but then simply get no treatment and be left to try and sort things out ourselves, which in some cases means further damage to our health (we will look at this in the next chapter). Sometimes the reasons given for not believing in our symptoms, or for believing us to be imagining them, are that what is happening to us doesn't fit the patterns that our doctors already understand. Sometimes, however, the reasons seem so bizarre that they can only be explained by an irrational but deeply embedded belief in the medical profession that women make things up to get attention or to express psychological problems.

It was definitely the case that: 'You can't possibly have this [ankylosing spondylitis]. You are far too young and you are the wrong sex. Only men get this.' It was ridiculous.

*Mary*

With the MS they said it was all psychosomatic, there's nothing the matter with you, go and see a psychiatrist or a psychologist and sort yourself out.

*Janet*

Women's health problems can also often be put down to hormonal disturbances. So often we can be told, 'It's your age', when complaining of health problems – that is to say, it's because we have started menstruating, are failing to menstruate, are pregnant, not pregnant, starting the menopause, and so on. It is strange that it can be so hard for real hormonal problems, such as premenstrual syndrome, to be taken seriously and yet so easy for other problems to be hung on this peg. There is in any case an ambivalence as to whether or not these explanations are really seen as physiological, since many doctors hold a thinly disguised belief that our hormones make us mad, or at best unreliable and confused.

Any history of mental health problems or symptoms perceived as related to sex are yet more reasons for doctors not to take us seriously:

> I was treated as an attention-seeker or a hypochondriac, mainly because I was abused from the age of 3 months until I was 16 or 17, and doctors tend to see that on your file. I was labelled, and no GP would send me to a specialist, that is until I had a problem with my knee and my GP thought it was a spontaneous fracture. The spina bifida was only diagnosed because a professor of orthopaedics happened to walk past when I was on a trolley and noticed that the way I was lying was wrong. So now, 30 years later, I am exonerated fully – but the pain and anguish they put me through ...
> 
> *Adele*

> When I was complaining of these pains the doctor was saying it was because I had been raped (which I hadn't been, I'd had a bad experience with my boyfriend). 'These problems are all in your mind.' He wouldn't listen to me at all, wouldn't examine me, just said I was a silly woman and put me on the Pill (to control the bleeding). I wouldn't say that I was backward in coming forward, but I'd started to wonder about my own sanity.
> 
> *Lesley*

If sexist attitudes in the medical profession stand in the way of women needing diagnosis and treatment, how much harder is it for working-class or black women, young or elderly women, still more prone to be judged unintelligent or untruthful? Labels of criminality or uncontrolled sexuality, sometimes attached to black people, may prevent health professionals seeing them as real people with real health problems. Juanita Cole, a black woman living in London, described in 1978 how her requests for an examination were repeatedly ignored by her doctor, until cancer spread throughout her reproductive organs – cancer which could have been easily detected and treated when she first reported symptoms:

> Aren't people like me supposed to get real sick? ... Must come as quite a shock to her [the nurse] that any of us has the nerve to up and die, or doesn't she think we do that either? Doctor there, he thinks we're so busy having babies we don't need, we can't never get sick ... and this woman, she thinks we're so busy taking free money from the dole, we don't have time to die ... I left [the surgery] almost hoping there was ... something seriously wrong, so maybe they would listen more closely to the next person.[15]

I am sure that doctors and all of us would prefer to believe such things could not happen now, nearly 20 years later. We can take some hope from Paris' experience of improving medical responses to pain caused by sickle-cell anaemia, and yet a letter from Sade came just as I was finishing this chapter, showing these racist attitudes very much alive and well in 1995:

> Earlier this year I had septic arthritis in my hip. Doctors doubted that I was in severe pain until they opened it up and found it full of infection. No one said sorry for doubting me. I developed lower back pain which temporarily paralysed me, was admitted to the same ward and, again, my pain was doubted by the nursing staff. The sister told me I was having too many pain

killers and that I wouldn't be going home with the drug because it was addictive. I said that, as a nurse, I was quite aware of the side effects. She never asked any of the other patients about their pain killers – just me, the only black patient on the ward. I wonder just what she was getting at.

*Sade*

Another pervasive and insidious area of discrimination is against women perceived as overweight, who are judged by doctors (and by other people) as being stupid, irresponsible and not worth listening to. Blaming women for causing their own illness, associating fatness with fecklessness and lack of self-control, presents a huge barrier to women (especially working-class women) getting appropriate treatment.

I'm hoping to try and lose a bit of weight. That definitely gives you more credibility. If you go with a grouch and you're slim, they're much more likely to take notice of you than if you're fat. Sounds silly but it's true, even if you go with a toothache.

*Patricia*

Every time it was my weight. If I went with a septic toe, it was my weight. My mum was a big lady and she was only four foot seven and she never ailed all her life. I'm not saying it helps, the weight, but it isn't the main cause.

*Bobby*

We are told these days that medical knowledge and technology enable early diagnosis and, therefore, early treatment for an ever-lengthening list of conditions. However, not all women will be able to benefit from this, if the health professionals they consult do not take their symptoms seriously. Doctors aim to save lives, yet those who make arbitrary and biased decisions about which of us to believe, may be making decisions about which of us will live or die. What right have they, entrusted with our health and our very lives, to decide that our blood, our pain or our tiredness are not significant or real? Do they know how completely they fail the women they should most be helping?

Fairly recently they've discovered a genetic link and I'm certain that a few women in my family had this condition. None of them had it diagnosed and they died young. My mother was only diagnosed shortly before her death, too late for the treatment to work. I feel really sad that these women had pretty miserable lives, feeling ill all the time; and that they didn't feel they could go to the doctor because the doctor would just say to them, 'It's because you're fat and you've got to lose weight.' My mother was humiliated so many times by doctors – because of her experience I went along somewhat better armed. She and other relatives could have had much happier, healthier and longer lives and I feel they were cheated, because underactive thyroid is a condition which has been known about and for which there's been a treatment for a long time. They were just poor women who lived in an area without good doctors, so nobody found out; and that haunts me still.

*Maggie*

## 6

# Passing the Buck: Who Is to Blame for Illness?

I don't feel like it was godly revenge or anything. I don't think it was written in my cards or my hands or my bones. No, it just happens. It happens to a hell of a lot of people.

*Harriet*

It's not as if your life is in a total cocoon from the outside world and you have total control over that cocoon. You're living on this planet and the planet's being destroyed.

*Jessie*

The consultant said to my friend once when she was sat having a cigarette, 'Now, what did I tell you about smoking, how it damages you?' and she said to him, 'What did you tell me about your radiotherapy and the damage it would do?'

*Lesley*

Most of us will ask the question 'Why me?' at some point, and many different concerns will affect how we think about this. Our understanding of the causes of our illness will make a difference to the way in which we incorporate it into our life and our world view. If we develop an illness as an adult, then our previous life experience and political, spiritual or other views will also influence how we interpret and respond to our condition. Equally, the fact of becoming ill, becoming a disabled person, is likely to alter our perspective on the world.

## 'Why me?': conflicting explanations for illness

Throughout women's accounts of life with illness runs an awareness of different explanations for illness, in particular of the conflict between explanations offered by medical professionals and alternatives which challenge these professional views. Debates about causes vary from one illness to another, but a common theme is the tension between individual and collective responsibility for illness (Lesley's friend, for example, questioned the right of her doctor to criticize her for smoking when her life was already threatened by the radiotherapy treatment he had given her). Women talking in this book have developed differing explanations, both medical and personal, for their illness. For some of us it may simply be a case of admitting that we don't know why, that doctors don't know why, that, as Harriet says, 'It just happens.' Whether we blame environmental pollution, the food we eat, the people we've slept with, childhood trauma or stress at work, all these explanations are inherently political because the identification of cause of illness is the first step in deciding how, as an individual or a society, we treat it.

Some illnesses, such as Paris' sickle-cell anaemia, are hereditary and the way they are passed on is fairly well understood:

> Mum and dad are both carriers so I was unlucky and got the full-blown disease. My sister was luckier and she's just a carrier. She has the trait so she can pass it on to her

children. I will pass it on to my children as well, they will be carriers, and if I married someone who had sickle cell then my children would definitely have the disease.

There are many other conditions where the genetic link is less well understood or is disputed. Medical opinions may conflict or change over time. For example, a woman quoted in Maternity Alliance's survey on disability was told she had a 50 per cent chance of passing on rheumatoid arthritis to her children. She avoided pregnancy for 11 years, only to find out eventually that this was not true.[1] The genetic element in diabetes has been the subject of much research over the years. It is passed on in a more complex way than something like sickle-cell anaemia, and there would appear to be important factors other than heredity determining whether any one individual becomes diabetic or not. It is a disease understood by many people to run in families, but there was no recent history of diabetes in my family, nor in those of other women with diabetes interviewed for this book:

> As soon as I was diagnosed, I wrote to my mum and dad and none of them had any history on either side to do with diabetes. My mum says my maternal grandmother died at a very early age, so she could have had it.
> *Kabita*

Angela's and Maureen's families both have some history of epilepsy, although Angela has been told that it isn't hereditary. Maureen's family believe her epilepsy to be the result of her having had meningitis only shortly after her birth.

Trying to work out where our illness comes from can also reveal previously unknown facts about our families, and may prove complicated or difficult. Janet has EDS, which is an inherited connective tissue disorder, but it was hard to trace back (and therefore to diagnose) as she was adopted as a baby. For Adele, piecing together an understanding of her illness has gone hand-in-hand with coming to understand her family, whom she refers to as 'a bunch of strangers held together by a name':

> I finally got the answer that no, it wasn't psychological and no, it wasn't physical trauma (i.e. something my mother did to me). I was born with spina bifida. Way, way back there was a spina bifida baby in my family. I know quite a bit of the family history because I got on well with my grandmother and she said I reminded her of my grandfather, who had similar health problems. I don't know my father, so I don't know if there was spina bifida in that family or not.

Some women with lupus know that other members of their family have it. This wasn't the case for Sade or Shirley, however, who both have other explanations for their illness:

> No, it's not in the family. The doctor said it was probably a virus that triggered everything off.
>
> *Sade*

> I wondered whether, if I'd been in a less stressful job, I might have had it more mildly, whether because the job (as a health visitor) was so very stressful, it came out worse.
>
> *Shirley*

Popular versions of medical research tend to focus on one simple explanation for any given illness. If a new possible cause is discovered by scientists, we may receive the impression that factors previously believed to be important are now discredited. Conflict is set up between, for instance, genetic and environmental explanations for breast cancer, and cholesterol, smoking or heredity as the main villain in causing heart disease. There may also be a confusion between long-term and short-term factors.

In reality, those of us who are ill are prepared for some degree of complexity or uncertainty in the reasons given for our illness. We accept that the precise course of illness will vary from one individual to another. Some of us have a strong feeling that one particular physical factor or life event has caused our illness, while others have settled for an explanation that incorporates a background factor, such as an inherited tendency or previous illness, with more immediate triggers, such as stress, overwork or a virus.

> I'm sure it [ME] was exacerbated by stress in the early days of trying to fight it, but I don't think anybody knows why they get anything, do they? In my last year at college I had two very bad doses of flu, and possibly one was glandular fever. I wonder if that's when the virus latched on in that way.
>
> *Francesca*

> I think the ankylosing spondylitis comes from my mother's side of the family. It's supposed to be hereditary, but some people, especially in the complementary medicine field, have said to me that it's stress-related, and I did have quite a stressful childhood. This word 'stress' is coming in for quite a lot of things, isn't it?
>
> *Mary*

Stress and viruses are commonly identified as the underlying cause of or trigger for an illness, to such an extent and for such a wide range of illnesses, that both terms are almost in danger of losing any serious meaning. Indeed, some people feel that if they visit the doctor and are told they have a virus, that this in fact means that the doctor doesn't know what the problem is, and can't or won't give any medication. The word 'stress' might be used by someone to describe their problems working in a highly paid, competitive job, which they neither enjoy much nor feel to be secure, and equally well by someone recently released from long-term psychiatric care, trying to deal with the benefits system, inadequate housing, social isolation and insecurity. Theories about stress management tend to focus on physiological mechanisms and effects rather than addressing the underlying reasons for stress (such as poverty or violence), which may in themselves be serious causes of ill health.

Knowing the underlying cause of our illness may be of less immediate importance for some of us than the recognition that we have become more ill than we might have done as a direct result of the medical profession's inadequate response. Jasmin had what she defines as chronic fatigue syndrome or post-viral syndrome and was ill for a couple of years, but is now almost entirely recovered. She was lucky in her doctor who identified it early and advised her to rest. Both the doctor and her acupuncturist told her that had it gone untreated for longer, it might have developed into ME, with much more serious consequences for her long-term health. Clare was not so lucky, however:

> I feel very angry that I wasn't believed and that their assumption was that it was all in the mind, because it meant that I went on for months trying to keep going and pull myself together when I should have been resting. I might have had a less serious illness and made a better recovery instead of still being ill now three years later. Why should I want to be ill, why should I want not to be able to work, or have relationships or anything?!
>
> *Clare*

For Lesley, the fact that treatment for cancer caused her current severe illness has radically changed her attitude to medicine and health. Anna knows that she got HIV from her sexual partner, but feels that this could have been prevented by better public information:

> It was through sex. It was at the beginning, 10 years ago, when people were talking about AIDS and I was thinking 'I don't do drugs, I can't get that. Can you get it from a fork?' And there I was sleeping with a man who had it but hadn't a clue that he had it, because he wasn't in any

of those 'high risk' groups. He died last year. I think that lack of information is still around now – women are still picking up HIV because they didn't believe they were at risk.

Jessie believes her ill health stems originally from medical prescription, but her experience also reflects how many different factors may affect our health:

> The first thing that went wrong with me was that I went on the Pill when I was 19, a big bloody mistake. I had no medical screening or anything, I just said to the doctor, 'I want to go on the Pill', and he said, 'Fine'. I got the most appalling symptoms: I got incredibly depressed, put on two stone in three months, was exhausted, couldn't keep awake. Before that I'd been really fit, I didn't get viruses or anything. I think the Pill damaged me on a permanent basis.

Jessie came off the Pill after five months and then immediately got thrush, for which she was misprescribed antibiotics. She soon developed glandular fever and chronic cystitis – a sign, she fears, of her lowered immunity as a result of the Pill and the antibiotics. After yet more antibiotics she started to become vulnerable to other viral infections. Against this background of less than perfect health, Jessie then started a new, very stressful job and after a while developed ME:

> It was very tiring and very pressurized, I was travelling all round the country. I didn't really have the resources for it. My immune system was definitely below par in the first place, I was in a relationship that wasn't nurturing me and I was working extremely hard. Another stress for me at the same time was digging up stuff about being abused as a child. Just before I got ill, I had a lot of conflict with my father, so there was also psychological stress affecting me.

Grace and Marlene, like many other women, see a clear relationship between childhood trauma and illness in adulthood:

> I am very interested in the way that women experience illness according to psychological trauma from childhood, because I've experienced that so specifically myself. For me, the deep seat of memory seems to be in the parts of the body where I was abused and where I am now developing problems. I think the difficulty is that it could be seen as if that makes it your own fault, that it's psychosomatic. I don't subscribe to those sort of attitudes to it.
>
> *Grace*[2]

> Sometimes when I'm feeling down I call myself the walking wounded. I think that I've come out sane up here (mind), but wounded down there (body), and I'd rather it was like that, because I couldn't bear anything to go wrong with my head. I was evacuated four times during the war, always onto people who didn't want me. They weren't cruel but they weren't kind either. One place the woman wouldn't allow us in the house except for meals. So I was always away from home, which was obviously where I wanted to be. Then when the war finished, three days after I came home, my father died from tuberculosis. A year later my mother committed suicide. That's what I mean, unhappy things happened to me, and I don't think you escape unscathed.
>
> *Marlene*

## 'It's your fault': blaming the victim

Causes of illness can therefore be seen as falling into various different categories, such as heredity, lifestyle, infection, stress or environment. As a society, however, we still seem to understand little about how these all interact. Breast cancer is an example of an illness where many different explanations are offered and hotly contested.[3]

> I had three sisters and I'm the only one that's ever had a lump on the breast, out of four girls, and my mother didn't have one either. A lot of people argue with me, but I do not think it is hereditary.
> *Woman at cancer support group*

In America, women with a family history of breast cancer have been encouraged to have healthy breasts removed as a preventive measure. Many doctors are so convinced that the disease is primarily a genetic one that they have blinded themselves to the drastic and brutal nature of this 'prevention'[4]. On the other hand, mounting evidence that links breast cancer with the use of pesticides, such as lindane, has not yet prevented the use of these in agriculture.[5] There are potentially many other illnesses over which the battle between genetics and environment could be fought, and the outcome of that conflict may have consequences for us all. Writer and disability activist, Anne Finger, describes one version of a future 'brave new world'[6]:

> I imagine a world where the air is thick and grey – although there are magnificent sunsets because of all the pollutants in the air – and embryos are routinely flushed from wombs and tested to be sure that they are resistant to radiation and toxicity – that is, that they do not have what has come to be known as the sicknesses of 'radia-

tion sensitivity' or 'toxicity intolerance' ... Maybe it would be better if the world just got blown up. I'll take the bang, not the whimper.[7]

We already live in a world where, rather than remove harmful agricultural pollutants from the environment, it is apparently preferable to chop off parts of women's bodies. How far can this approach be taken? How many parts of our bodies are to be categorized as useless or dangerous to us? Fixing on the breast itself as the problem, rather than the pesticides or nuclear radiation[8] which harm it, is victim-blaming taken to ridiculous extremes – surely only a few small steps away from Finger's nightmare vision.

There are other factors believed by some to increase the likelihood of breast cancer, such as high consumption of animal fat or alcohol, or use of a combined contraceptive pill at an early age. All these are debated and have a variety of implications for individuals and society as a whole. We need to look not only at the apparent original cause of disease, however, but at the reasons for unequal survival rates once it is diagnosed.

Black American women diagnosed with breast cancer die, on average, far more quickly than their white counterparts with the same disease.[9] Women need information to keep themselves healthy where possible, information about diet, alcohol and other things over which there is some degree of personal control. However by focusing primarily on individual behaviour, society ignores the effects of poverty or oppression, and adds insult to injury in blaming the few for the illnesses caused by the actions of the many. Those with least power and control over their lives receive the lion's share of the blame for their ill health, while doctors, manufacturers of drugs and pesticides, producers of energy and weapons, and others with the wealth and power to make changes escape scot free.

Many of us collude in this unjust victim-blaming because we want to live, we fear death and wish to believe that we can by our own actions protect ourselves and those we love from harm. More and more evidence is nowadays available to us that poverty causes more ill health than any other single factor[10]. It takes only a minimal amount of common sense to see how inadequate, cold or damp housing, long hours and stress at work, low pay, lack of food, insecurity and violence take their toll on men's and women's bodies. Similarly, the effects of environmental pollution are daily drawn to our attention. Yet all the time those of us living in wealthier countries or communities search ever more desperately for small-scale, individual solutions.

The idealized, healthy body, talked about in Chapter 1, has come to symbolize not only strength, beauty and sexuality, but our individual degree of control over our lives. Whole groups of people (such as women and disabled people) are often described in this culture as not being in control of their bodies, as being at the mercy of biology. Nevertheless, the trend towards individual responsibility for and control over health, means that the ideal body is presented as something within the grasp of each or any of us – if we would but try hard enough. In the past, impairment or illness was seen in some societies as a sign of divine displeasure, a visible punishment for some sin. The wheel has perhaps come full circle as now if we appear ill, fat or even old, it is seen as caused by something we have done wrong. We have eaten the wrong food or too much of it, smoked cigarettes, drunk too much alcohol or coffee, failed to take enough exercise or enough rest.

Our lack of control over our health and environment, together with the scale of the problems which threaten them, make us despair. Government policies in Britain and America have increased poverty and destroyed local public services. The companies which produce the food we eat, which affect the quality of the air we breathe and the water we drink, operate on a worldwide scale and amid such secrecy that few of us feel able to understand the issues in detail or to challenge their policies and behaviour. So, rather than campaigning for the right of everyone to safe, affordable, healthy food, we limit ourselves to controlling as far as possible what we put in our own bodies. We purchase water filters rather than campaigning for free and equal access for all to clean water. Those of us who can afford vitamin pills, filters and good quality, fresh food purchase every day better health and longer life than those who are too poor to buy these things.

It is hard to live with this knowledge, however, and so we eagerly latch on to explanations for illness which lay responsibility at the door of the individual. We stigmatize and learn to hate people who are ill. Once ill ourselves, we face a choice between living with self-loathing or accepting only too late the limitations of the culture of blame.

> When I first had cervical cancer people's attitudes were terrible – one male colleague said to me, 'Well, it's your fault, because you only get cervical cancer if you go with loads of men.' The number of women this has upset because they've only ever had one partner!
>
> *Vicky*

It was believed not long ago that a lot of sexual activity made women more prone to changes in the cervix leading to cancer. More recently a correlation has been found between the incidence of cervical cancer and the number of sexual partners the woman's *partner* has had. However irrelevant, the association of cervical cancer with promiscuity in women persists in many people's minds. Similar to this faulty attachment of blame over cancer is the demonization of women as carriers of AIDS, touched on earlier. Current medical knowledge tells us that female-to-male transmission of the HIV virus through sexual intercourse is extremely difficult without the presence of some other factor, such as another infection. It is men who can easily spread the virus to women, rather than the other way round. This is not, in turn, to demonize men and male sexuality, but simply to note that we live in a women-blaming society – a society in which men are discouraged from taking responsibility for their sexuality, and in which public beliefs about AIDS bear little or no relation to biological reality.

## Passing the Buck

Myalgic encephalomyelitis or ME is another illness hedged about with medical and public misconceptions. As a fairly new illness, it has received much media attention and given rise to speculation about causes and treatment. The vast majority of people diagnosed with it are women (though it may be true that men with ME don't get diagnosed because it is seen as a women's disease) and this may be the reason for the many peculiar myths that have developed around it, and for doctors and many other people failing to take it seriously.

> There is a myth about yuppy women in their 30s wanting it all and overdoing it, and it serves the poor dears right. They'd feel better if they got pregnant – all this nonsense.
>
> *Francesca*

> I heard this psychiatrist going on about how people with ME were all women in their 30s who were unhappy with their relationships. It worries me that it's also seen so exclusively as a middle-class disease. I'm convinced there are working-class women with ME in psychiatric wards whose physical symptoms haven't been taken seriously.
>
> *Jessie*

> There are so many myths about it, like the one that says you can cure it by having a cold bath every day.
>
> *Clare*

The fact that the public face of the ME sufferer is a middle-class one, may tell us only that the media is more concerned with the experience of middle-class than with working-class women, or, perhaps, that middle-class women can more easily assert themselves in the face of an unsympathetic and disbelieving Health Service, so as to get a diagnosis. The effect of doctors and journalists characterizing this illness as one affecting 'yuppy' women, women who will have had greater choice than others about work, education and children, is once again to blame women for getting ill. When poor women get ill, they are blamed for their irresponsibility or stupidity. When middle-class women get ill, they are told it is because they are self-indulgent or have unrealistic expectations of life. The emergence of such a new illness could lead us to ask questions about how healthy our world is. Instead society focuses on women's 'unreasonable' desires for fulfilment in work, relationships and family life.

The language of conflict, separation and blame which society uses to discuss illness is in itself confusing and harmful. Thinking and talking about illness as a separate and evil part of our person puts enormous barriers in the way of those of us who live with illness long term, and who must therefore find some positive way of integrating it into our personality and identity. We learn instead to hate our illness, and sometimes also the treatments or equipment which go with it or come to represent it.

Doctors, researchers and medical charities constantly talk about the fight against cancer, diabetes or arthritis, and the hope that we can eradicate major diseases from the earth. Yet how does society confront or experience illness except as it is manifested in people? The confusion between a disease and the people who have that disease is evident when medical professionals and health planners discuss resources for health care. At a conference I attended once, a leading diabetes specialist spoke about the abundance of money available for AIDS research and the lack of money for work on diabetes (because, he joked, AIDS involves sex and diabetes does not).[11] The people with diabetes in the audience were being invited to lend credibility to professional concerns and jealousy. We were implicitly being described as respectable, deserving people, unlike people who get AIDS.

In real life, illness is no respecter of divisions between medical specialities. A person with diabetes, asthma or MS may also be a person with AIDS. All of us, but especially those of us already ill, need good quality, well-resourced, coordinated health care. Besides our specialist care for our illness, we need such things as properly functioning accident and emergency services, well-informed and flexible maternity services and affordable dental care. We are not well served by squabbles over resources and by doctors who are only interested in our arthritis or sickle-cell anaemia rather than our whole person and well-being.

## 'A popular way of thinking': the future without illness

Scientists talk about a future free from various diseases, perhaps free from all disease. Is it possible to talk about eradicating certain types of illness without, in fact, saying that we want to eradicate people who have that disease? Are we not saying that the world would be a better place without people with sickle-cell anaemia, without people with diabetes, asthma or heart disease? The increasing pace of genetic research raises worrying possibilities for those of us who fail to match up to society's ideal.

> The race for identifying the genetic causes of disease is another problem isn't it? It's all geared towards a time when those things can be 'bred out', which is exactly what Hitler wanted to do. At the time of Hitler, it was a very popular way of thinking, racial cleansing was perfectly acceptable. It seems to be coming round again, but being sold now as science ideology rather than racial ideology.
> 
> *Grace*

The debate between genetics and environment or nature and nurture, which resurfaces every so often, is fundamental to what kind of society we think we are. Which side of the line we decide to come down on determines how we organize resources and how we treat people. Some scientists are currently claiming to find genetic markers not only for particular physical or mental illnesses, but also for homosexuality, obesity and violent or criminal behaviour. These findings are hailed as advances for humanity, because they may make it possible to 'treat' such deviations from what is regarded as desirable or normal. Gene replacement therapy is the latest area of research into which much research money is being poured. In theory, this could enable doctors in the future to alter the genetic material of embryos identified as carrying some particular illness.[12] So rather than kill 'defective' embryos, we could just fix them up, just get rid of the sickle-cell anaemia, potential violence or the likelihood of being a fat person.

These possibilities raise huge questions about the nature of individuality and the rights of individuals versus those of society. There are, in fact, only a few diseases (such as cystic fibrosis or sickle-cell anaemia) which have only one genetic marker, where the hereditary process is straightforward. Many others, as far as we know, have more than one, besides having apparent causes other than heredity. We do not know what other effects might arise from this meddling with our genes. If it had been possible in 1959, when I was in my mother's womb, to change the genes which contained the possibility of my developing diabetes in adulthood, would I still be the same person in every other way? If not, whose decision should it have been to alter me? Who is to decide what is normal, what is good or bad? Do we want a world without fat people, gay men and lesbians, a world perhaps without people with red hair?

Huge changes have been taking place in the British Health Service in recent years, and the likelihood is of still more changes in the years ahead. Even if genetic science is not used to alter people, the identification of people likely to develop certain diseases during their lives could be useful to planners and providers of health care. Right-wing politicians would like to see the British health-care system nearer to the American model, dependent more on private insurance than on taxation. Genetic screening could render many people uninsurable from birth, leaving them without health care. In a society placing increasing responsibility on the individual to maintain their own health through a 'good' lifestyle, many of us could spend even more years living with special rules and constraints, and living with the spectre of moral failure and stigma if we finally become ill.

Ever greater possibilities are opened up for identifying some people as undeserving of health care and others as too expensive for society to cope with. In both Britain and America, the debate about who should get health care is becoming much more explicit. Politicians (and some doctors) tell us that the demand for health care is infinite. By encouraging us to believe that the health needs of all can never be met, they hope to enlist our support for decreasing public expenditure on health. It is essential that we challenge theories which obscure the real causes of illness, and that we are not lured into more victim-blaming, into seeing other's rights to health care as conflicting with our own.

## 'Men make me bloody angry': getting political

The experience of living with illness in a culture which does not value ill and disabled people has influenced the way that many of the women in this book think about the world, politics and health. Some of us have always been resistant to mainstream culture and beliefs, others have been politicized or changed by becoming ill.

For some of us, as we have seen, therapies such as acupuncture, homoeopathy, aromatherapy or diet have provided an alternative or antidote to conventional medicine. Fundamental to most complementary therapies is a holistic approach, treating the whole person as opposed to individual organs or parts of the body, as Marlene says of practitioners in these fields, 'They take an interest in you as a person.' So, of course, do the best nurses and doctors, but most are prevented from doing so by lack of time and training. We know from our own experience of our bodies that psychological and physical factors interact with each other, and it can be an enormous relief to find a professional to talk to who recognizes this. Complementary therapies can also be especially important for women, because they take more account of our female hormonal system and how this affects our health. Another advantage is the lack of unwanted side effects. Because acupuncture or homoeopathic treatment, for example, will always take into account our whole body, we do not have to worry that by treating one part of our body we may be damaging another.

Complementary medicine can offer a radical challenge to the culture of victim-blaming as a result of this holistic approach. It offers the possibility of a more equal relationship between practitioner and patient, one that is realistic about the multiple stresses on our health. It fits in well with a view of the world that incorporates the desire for a healthy environment, and rejects the harm done to people in the name of science and technology. It does, however, have its own limitations, the most obvious of which is that it is mainly available privately. Marlene and Anna have both found some treatment available within the Health Service, but this is still rare (due to the dismissive attitude towards alternative medicine by most medical professionals). Though many practitioners have sliding fee scales, for most women low benefit or wage levels would not allow more than a token payment. So, in effect, complementary therapies become yet another way for a very few of us to improve or manage our health.

Perhaps partly because they operate mainly within the realm of individual choice, many complementary therapists have also developed a very individualistic approach to health. Their holism does not often extend beyond the boundaries of the single body and mind, and they present health as being totally within our individual control. Just as with conventional preventive medicine, we are given a set of rules to live by, such as avoiding alcohol, cigarettes or various kinds of food. Once again the blame for illness can be laid on our shoulders if we do not do the right things. The much clearer understanding that exists within complementary medicine of the links between physical and mental well-being can also lead to undue pressure to think positively all the time. It becomes a duty to have our emotional house completely in order. The most extreme version of this has been perhaps in relation to cancer, in the idea of the 'cancer personality', the idea that cancer is a result of an unhappy attitude to life. Audre Lorde challenged this concept at the end of the 1970s, though it persists today in both conventional and alternative attitudes to cancer treatment:

> ... looking on the bright side of things is a euphemism used for obscuring certain realities of life, the open consideration of which might prove threatening or dangerous to the status quo. Last week I read a letter from a doctor in a medical magazine which said that no truly happy person ever gets cancer ... for a moment this letter hit my guilt button. Had I really been guilty of the crime of not being happy in this best of all possible infernos?[13]

Practising positive thinking and having knowledge of ways to treat our own illness can empower us to take back control of our health and our bodies, but we can also be distracted from attending to what is going on around us. Political movements, such as feminism or the disabled people's movement, are important precisely because they help us to focus on what is wrong with the world rather than the individual.

> The government and councils are pretty damning towards the disabled and it needs somebody to shout. I'm not afraid of shouting. I've been a bit of a rebel, but haven't done anything magic. I've been reading the book

*Growing Old Disgracefully* and I couldn't agree more! I'm all for the various women's movements. It'll be slow getting there, but what isn't for God's sake?

*Angela*

The thing that I've become too is a feminist. Men make me bloody angry. It's not that I don't like men, but they're in charge of everything and they're making such a mess of it, just lousing everything up.

*Marlene*

Both feminism and disability politics can be profoundly liberating for us as individuals. They tell us that we are not second-rate, we are not the problem, that society is at fault in the way that it treats us. The women's health movement was an important strand of feminism during the 1970s and 80s, and through it I and many other women have been helped to a greater understanding of our health and biology, and to a belief in our right to control what happens to our own bodies. The very early days of women's groups learning to use speculums to examine their cervixes have now become something of a joke, but those women were challenging the misogyny and inaccuracy of medical ideas about women's anatomy and biology.[14]

The disability movement has mounted a more fundamental challenge to the right of the medical profession to define what is the matter with us and to decide what needs fixing in our bodies. By arguing that disabled people's problems stem more from discrimination than from their individual impairments, this movement has also made it possible for many disabled men and women to feel good about themselves and their bodies for the first time. Our sense of self-worth is essential to our survival and anything that strengthens it is a blow struck for our freedom.

Another important source of support for women living with illness, both practically and politically, has been the self-help movement. In Britain and America (and increasingly in the rest of Europe and worldwide), there are now self-help groups for almost every conceivable medical condition or other problem. The development of these groups in the past couple of decades has stemmed partly from the need to find alternatives to medical views, and partly from the recognition of the comfort and strength we gain from knowing that another person has shared our particular experience and understands it. An organizer of a support group for women with breast cancer said the first question asked by every woman who comes to the group is, 'Have you had a mastectomy yourself?'

> I've got a friend who I met when I was pregnant, who became diabetic. We were both struck down by something during pregnancy that we've got to live with for the rest of our lives, and I think that promotes a sort of kinship. It's just nice to know that it happens to other people as well.
>
> *Maggie*

> I often feel quite cheerful when I meet other people who say they think they've got the same thing as I have, or that a friend of theirs has or whatever. I feel a lot of empathy.
>
> *Francesca*

Many, if not all of the women in this book would describe themselves as some sort of feminist. Francesca, Clare, Grace and Angela are or have been actively involved in disability politics, and some others of us are more passive members of disabled people's organizations. Several of us have also been involved in self-help or support groups for people with the same condition as ourselves. Jessie puts much of her time and energy into an ME support group, as does Lesley into RAGE (Radiotherapy Action Group Exposure) and Janet into the Ehlers-Danlos Syndrome Support Group. Some of these groups focus on offering support and information to members, while others also campaign for more research funds to be allocated, or more generally for better public and government recognition of their particular illness and the problems associated with it.

All these and other political movements (such as anti-racist, anti-poverty or environmental campaigning) defy the attempts of those in power to define society's problems and to blame them on the rest of us. However, they each also have their limitations. Several women in this book expressed some dissatisfaction with the orthodoxy of belief in the disabled people's movement, which sometimes seems to exclude people who do not feel positive about their illness or impairment. Women who do not have the energy or desire to get involved in high-profile political action can also be left feeling helpless or inadequate.

> The local disabled people's organization seems to ignore people whose disability has a strong medical component, and they talk as if you're a traitor to the cause if you want to disguise the fact that you've had an arm amputated. I don't think they have the right to say whether or not you wear a prosthesis or have operations to make you walk again. People are different and should make their own decision.
>
> *Eleanor*

> I think disabled people should really speak up, but it needs to be got across that there are some people who are disabled and ill, and some people who are disabled but not ill.
>
> *Adele*

However, even those of us who are not always sure about the approach taken by some disabled people's organizations know that, as Eleanor says, 'If the more militant people get changes then I'll benefit.'

The main problem with much of feminist politics, and also with the self-help movement, is that too many women are excluded. National self-help organizations still mainly benefit white people, and though this may partly be because black people choose to organize differently around health issues, it is also down to a failure to recognize differences between people with the same illness. Women with the same illness, but from very different backgrounds, will of course have many physical experiences in common and may get much comfort from speaking to one another. However, it is also essential to recognize that both our own attitudes to our illness and the support we get from the medical profession and elsewhere will vary enormously according to our class, race, age or sexuality. Self-help groups can be complacent in their assumption that they are open to everyone with a particular illness, and many exclude people by not recognizing their different experience and needs.

We are living in the 1990s with the legacy of the failure of the women's movement in the 70s and 80s to include and represent black women, working-class women, lesbians, disabled women and many others. I believe that all women are now disadvantaged by a continuing inability to find common ground among all our differences. One of the ways in which women continue to be excluded from groups and organizations is by being made to feel that they do not belong or do not measure up. Models of behaviour and belief have been created by both feminist and disability politics, which in many ways challenge an oppressive establishment, but which also serve as impossible ideals for us to live up to. If we cannot juggle work, family and political campaigning then we feel ourselves to be second-rate. Many feminists and disabled activists have, I believe, fallen into the trap of believing that, in order to be strong and powerful, we must transcend or ignore our biology and physical reality. So, those of us who cannot always feel good about our ill bodies, feel ourselves to fall short not only of society's image of womanhood but also of the model of a 'good feminist' or 'good disabled person'.

## 'Just poor women': remembering our common humanity

When I started thinking about this book, I knew that I did not want to write only about the views and experience of women like myself, and I have tried to speak to women of different ages, races and classes. I know that there are many voices which are absent, voices of women whom I could not have reached without more time, more resources and more understanding of their experience. Each of us whose lives you have read about here, however extreme the problems we have faced, are conscious that we are more fortunate than many others. Over and over again in their interviews women said such things as: 'But I know how to fight for things', 'I'm lucky to have a good doctor', 'I know how to use a library', 'I can read English', 'I got information through work.' Some of us had fewer resources than others to help us in our struggle, but all of us are painfully aware of how much harder still our experience could have been. We know how much more difficult it is for the many women out there who have far less knowledge, power or control over their lives than we do.

Even those of us who feel reasonably secure and comfortable cannot help but be aware of the changes that have taken place in Britain's economy and social system. Even those of us who have suffered little so far from these changes have fears for ourselves and for others, as we see inequality grow and collective support for those who need it diminish with every year that passes. And this is just in Britain, still absurdly wealthy despite a stagnating economy and growing poverty. This book has not even tried to address the lives of women living with illness in parts of the world where there is not enough food, let alone enough health care.

So in wealthy, privileged, liberal, democratic Britain, there are many women living with the same illnesses as those discussed in this book, but who also have learning difficulties or other more severe physical impairments. There are women living with long-term illness in prison, in psychiatric care or in old people's homes; women living with illness on the streets or in violent families; women who can't read and write or who don't speak English; women who have no legal status in this country or who are just too poor or have been too badly treated to believe that they deserve any better. For all these reasons there are thousands of women with the same health needs as those in this book but who get none of these needs met. They have little or no say about what medication they are on, no means of redress if doctors fail to treat them correctly, no control over their diet or day-to-day activity, no access to information about alternative treatments.

The longer I live with diabetes and appreciate the good health I still have, the more conscious I am of the good things in life: of the sun on my skin, the roof over my head, food and wine shared with friends or a walk with my dog by a river. And so the more intolerable it is that so many other women are more ill than they need be, live shorter lives than need be and live in more pain or distress than they need do because they lack the treatment, money or freedom to enable them to be better. It is because life is good that injustice and inequality matter. Once we know the value of what we have, then it matters that others don't have the same. On every good day that I have, when diabetes is no more than a nuisance and I have the energy to do most of what I have planned, there is perhaps another woman out there, very like me, who could be having as good a day but is not – because she is on the wrong insulin, doesn't understand her diet, is living in a damp house, has no money to buy good food, no one to help with her children, no place in which she can safely take exercise, no comfortable place to sit.

Our physical existence enables us to feel both great pain and great pleasure. Pain and illness are part and parcel of being human. When I was young, my mother told me how she had wept when I was born because the fact of my birth meant that I would die. We cannot have life without death, and if we love life we can embrace it in its totality, including its end. To believe that perfect physical health is normal and a right, rather than a gift and a bonus, is to set ourselves up for failure and self-hatred and to create a society which fears and despises many of its own members.

We need desperately to find a way to be less afraid of illness, to accept people who live with illness and impairment as normal, viable and valuable human beings, but at the same time to reject the more insane industrial, economic and medical practices which cause so much illness. Why should we accept as inevitable illness caused or exacerbated by medical mistakes or negligence, which could have been prevented if we had been believed or if we had more control over our lives and more resources to help us thrive? Why should we accept with equanimity all the illness, pain and premature death caused by pollution, damp housing or starvation?

Maggie is haunted by the deaths of her mother and other relatives who were ill for much of their lives – 'They were just poor women in an area without good doctors, so nobody found out' – and as I finish this book they haunt me too. There are other ghosts: Lesley's friend who died from radiotherapy injuries, or Juanita Cole who spoke about her cancer in 1978, but of whose later life or death I have no record. During these days of sitting at a computer, sifting through piles of words, it is these absent women who hover at my shoulder, their silence filling the room, occupying my mind.

I know too that for every woman who reads this and who may find it useful, many more will never see it. To all those women struggling with illness whose words and lives are not shown here, though this may not be written about you, it is written for you as much as for any of us. We whose experience makes up this book know that you are out there and that, wherever, whoever you are, you feel some of the same things we feel. We know that you matter. To anyone else reading this, remember that, but for whatever accident, fate or grace you believe in, any of the women in this book, any of those other, absent women out there could be me, or could be you.

Veronica Marris
5 Brundretts Road, Manchester, M21 9DA, tel: 0161 860 5625

9/9/96

Dear Tyrrell,
Here are books — have enclosed a note for Peter + Dolores in theirs. Thanks for phoning. Will send more news of Lisa in a while. All best, Veronica

## Passing the Buck

> No man is an island, entire of itself, but a part of the whole; ... any man's death diminishes me for I am a part of mankind; and therefore never send to know for whom the (funeral) bell tolls; it tolls for thee.
>
> *John Donne, seventeenth-century poet, writing in the midst of a serious illness*[15]

Illness and disability can affect anyone, no matter how well we look after ourselves. To understand that we have only partial control over our health is not to despair but to accept the limitations of human power, to subdue a little our craving for control, and lose a little of our fear.

> I don't want to die, but since I accepted the fact that I probably will, I am more at peace. It's as if my energy had been used up denying the reality of my own impending death and, when I stopped struggling against the idea, I suddenly felt free. I could begin to think about living again.
>
> *Woman talking about facing cancer*[16]

We live in a world in which people desperately want to believe that pain and weakness, old age and, ultimately, death can be avoided by means of operations, diets, positive thinking, anti-ageing creams or workouts in the gym; a world in which illness is a sign of moral failure; a world which imagines some of our lives to be not worth living because physical strength and material achievement are the only goals to aim for, the only gods to be worshipped. The experience of living with illness offers us instead a chance to realize our own essential and intrinsic value and that of others; it offers us the knowledge that all lives are worth living.

# References

## Introduction

1. Anne Finger, *Past Due: a story of disability, pregnancy and birth*, Women's Press, London, 1991.
2. Maggie O'Kane, 'The X Files', *Guardian*, 6 July 1995; *Deadly Experiments*, Twenty Twenty TV, shown on Channel 4 on 6 July 1995.
3. See Ivan Illich, *Limits to Medicine, Medical Nemesis: The Expropriation of Health*, Penguin, London, 1990 (originally published by Marion Boyars, 1976).

## 1: Feeling Different: Isolation, Invisibility and Identity

1. Audre Lorde, *The Cancer Journals*, Sheba, London, 1985.
2. 'Women Like Us: Survey on the Needs and Experiences of HIV Positive Women', Positively Women, London, October 1994.
3. See, for instance, Sheila Kitzinger's well-known *Freedom & Choice in Childbirth*, Penguin, London, 1988; and Boston Women's Health Collective, *The New Our Bodies Ourselves* (ed. Angela Phillips and Jill Rakusen, UK edition), Penguin, London, 1989. Both books mention disability and various illnesses, but mainly in relation to prenatal screening for impairment in the foetus.
4. Ntozake Shange, *Spell # 7*, Methuen, Reed Books, London, 1985 (in association with the Women's Playhouse Trust).
5. Until the early 1980s, people with insulin-dependent diabetes used insulin extracted from the pancreas of pigs or cows. Since then it has become possible to genetically engineer insulin in the laboratory so

that its structure is the same as insulin found in humans. This is now what most people use, but during the last decade some people have experienced very disabling side effects when changing from animal to human insulin.
6. Positively Women, op. cit.

## 2: Feeling Useful: Work, Roles and Contributing to Society

1. See, for instance, on sick-leave policy in the NHS, Andrew Cole, 'Getting sick of ill nurses', *Guardian*, 4 May 1994.
2. See Kat Duff, *The Alchemy of Illness*, Virago, London, 1994, pp. 4–9 on the contrasting worlds of illness and health.
3. See, for example, Lesley Doyal, *What Makes Women Sick: Gender and the Political Economy of Health*, Macmillan, London, 1995, pp. 10–14; Kate Figes, *Because Of Her Sex: the myth of equality for women in Britain*, Macmillan, London, 1994. See pp. 145–46 regarding women, poverty and the use of health care.
4. Jenny Morris, *Independent Lives?: Community Care and Disabled People*, Macmillan, London, 1993. See pp. 82–4 for Audrey's story and that of Vicky who experienced violence at the hands of her woman partner, also pp. 67–8 and 115–16 for other experiences of abuse in residential care or by home carers.

## 3: Strange Attitudes: Coping with People Coping with Us

1. 'Living with Sickle Cell Anaemia', *Women's Health*, issue 20, November 1993, from Women's Health, 52 Featherstone Street, London, EC1R 8RT.
2. Audre Lorde, op. cit.

## 4: Not a Real Woman?: Love, Sex and Families

1. Positively Women, op. cit.
2. Audre Lorde, op. cit.; and on prostheses see also Dr Cathy Read,

*Preventing Breast Cancer: the politics of an epidemic*, Pandora, London, 1995, pp 28–32.
3. For more discussion of disabled women, sexuality and motherhood, see Jenny Morris, *Pride Against Prejudice*, Women's Press, London, 1991; Jenny Morris, *Able Lives*, Women's Press, London, 1989; Meg Goodman, 'Mothers Pride and others Prejudice: a survey of disabled mothers' experiences of maternity', Maternity Alliance Disability Working Group, London, 1994.
4. Mary Shackle, 'I thought I was the only one: report of a conference Disabled People, Pregnancy and Early Parenthood', Maternity Alliance Disability Working Group, London, 1994.
5. See Beverley Bryan, Stella Dadzie and Suzanne Scarfe, *The Heart of the Race*, Virago, London, 1985, pp. 100–107; various articles on Depo Provera in Sue Sullivan (ed.), *Women's Health: A Spare Rib Reader*, Pandora, London, 1987; Stephen Trombley, *The Right to Reproduce: A History of Coercive Sterilisation*, Weidenfeld & Nicolson, London, 1988; a recent example given me by a deaf women's health group was of a woman discovering, after months of trying to conceive, that her doctor had given her Depo Provera injections without even asking if she needed or wanted contraception!
6. Mary Schackle, op. cit.
7. Meg Goodman, op. cit.
8. Positively Women, op. cit.
9. Puerperal psychosis is the most extreme and easily identifiable form of post-natal depression. It is rare (occurring in up to 1 per 1,000 births) but serious. See Ann Oakley, *Women Confined: Towards a Sociology of Childbirth*, Martin Roberton, Oxford, 1980.
10. Report from Women and Diabetes National Meeting, Manchester, March 1992, organized by Women & Diabetes Network (contact through British Diabetic Association).

# 5: Biting the Hand that Feeds Us: Dealing with the Doctors

1. See Boston Women's Health Collective, op. cit., pp. 607–38, on the politics of women in health care.
2. Protasia Torkington in *Healthy & Wise: an essential health handbook for black women*, (ed.) Melba Wilson, Virago, London, 1994, pp. 18–25.
3. Positively Women, op. cit.
4. This became possible under the Access to Health Records Act (1991), although the Act was not retrospective and so only relates to information recorded from 1991 onwards. Under the Data Protection Act (1984) patients also have rights to see information

## References

held on computer and it is possible in the future that data protection legislation will also cover non-computerized records. In both cases doctors retain rights to withold information if they consider it could harm the patient.

5. Positively Women, op. cit.
6. ibid.
7. See, for instance, Lesley Doyal, op. cit. p. 17; and regarding the invisibility of black women in medical research, see Jenny Douglas, 'Black women's health matters' in Helen Roberts (ed.) *Women's Health Matters*, Routledge, London, 1992.
8. See Marge Berer and Sunanda Ray, *Women and HIV/AIDS: an international resource book*, Pandora, London, 1993; and Lesley Doyal, op. cit., p. 17, regarding AIDS research.
9. Audre Lorde, op. cit.
10. Paula Fenton Thomas, in Melba Wilson, op. cit., pp. 104–12.
11. See also John Illman, 'Mark of the Wolf', *Guardian*, 5 April 1995, about Julie Dennis, a woman with lupus who had difficulties getting diagnosed and was told off by a doctor for complaining about too many different symptoms at once!
12. Community Health Councils were set up in Britain in 1974 to represent patients' rights and views within the Health Service. There is a CHC for each health district, with members elected from the local population and paid staff providing support and information to the public.
13. See Boston Women's Health Collective, op. cit., pp. 625–35, on suggestions for getting a better deal out of the system.
14. 'London Hospitals Study', *British Medical Journal*, 30 April 1993; and also see 'Coronary Heart Disease: Are Women Special?', report from National Forum for Coronary Heart Disease Prevention, London, 1994; Maureen Freely, 'Heart Failure', *Guardian*, 24 November 1994.
15. Thomas Cottle, *Black Testimony, the voices of Britain's West Indians*, Wildwood House, London, 1978.

# 6: Passing the Buck: Who Is to Blame for Illness?

1. Meg Goodman, op. cit.
2. See Kat Duff, op. cit., for more discussion of remembering in the body with reference to ME.
3. Dr Cathy Read, op. cit.; Sharon Batt, *Patient No More*, Scarlet Press, London, 1995.
4. See description by a medical student of a surgeon in theatre saying,

'All women should have prophylactic (preventive) mastectomies. Breasts are pathological', Nuria Martinez Alier, in newsletter of Women in Medicine (organization for women doctors and medical students), January 1995.
5. Dr Cathy Read, op. cit.; Campaign Pack from Women's Environmental Network (Aberdeen Studios, 22 Highbury Grove, London N52EA); Laura Potts and Mary Twomey, 'From Private Shame to Public Campaign', *Health Matters*, issue 22, summer 1995.
6. William Shakespeare, *The Tempest*, 'Oh brave new world that has such people in it!'; Title of Aldous Huxley's book (written in 1932) describing a world where reproduction is controlled and organized by the state, with only some people allowed to reproduce, embryos developed in test tubes and engineered to fit pre-determined roles in society.
7. Anne Finger, op. cit.
8. Kat Duff, op. cit., pp. 44–5.
9. Lesley Doyal, op. cit., p.13
10. Chris Mihill, 'Public Enemy Number One', *Guardian*, 2 May 1995; 'Tackling Inequalities in Health: an agenda for action', (ed.) Michaela Benzeval, Len Judge and Margaret Whitehead, Kings Fund, 1995; *Inequalities in Health: the Black Report and the Health Divide*, Peter Townsend, Nick Davidson and Margaret Whitehead, Penguin, London, 1988.
11. British Diabetic Association Glucose Control Workshop, October 1993.
12. At the present time this is still illegal.
13. Audre Lorde, op. cit.
14. On inaccurate anatomy textbooks, see Jocelyn Wogan-Browne in newsletter of Women in Medicine, op. cit.
15. John Donne, *Meditations*.
16. Boston Women's Health Collective, op. cit., p.581.

# Biographies of the Women Interviewed

There now follow some brief details about the 27 women with whom I conducted full-length interviews. The book also includes quotations or information from three women who spoke to me when I visited cancer support groups, and also some from women I have met in other groups or have spoken to casually.

Half the women interviewed are living on benefits or a comparably low income; somewhere between a third and a half grew up in working-class or low-income families; and over two-thirds either have a degree (quite often taken as a mature student) or a qualification in a discipline such as nursing, teaching or social work. Six out of the 27 are black, the rest are white. In terms of age, exactly one third are in their 30s, one third in their 40s, five in their 20s and four aged between 50 and 65. Two women are lesbian and two mentioned having relationships with both men and women, the rest I know or guess to be heterosexual. Only 11 women have children (see more details in Chapter 4). Thirteen live alone, though two of these have partners who do not live with them.

**Adele** is 31, white and lives on her own. She was born with spina bifida and several other conditions which have deteriorated in adulthood and cause her to be in pain much of the time. She gets disability benefits and has social services carers. She spends her time looking after her house and many pets and likes to get out as often she can.

**Anna** is nearing 40, white, has been HIV positive for nine years, but so far has stayed healthy. She lives with her son and works in the voluntary sector. She says she is enjoying life and looking forward to her future.

**Angela** is a retired dental surgeon in her 60s, white, and has had epilepsy since her teens. She is divorced with four grown-up children of whom one son lives with her. In recent years she has developed diabetes and asthma. She has a busy life, including being the chair of her local disabled people's association.

**Bobby** is 48, white and has diabetes, asthma, heart disease and arthritis. She lives with her husband, who is also disabled, and three daughters; another daughter is married with three children. She used to do voluntary work at a local community centre, but has recently suffered a heart attack and can't do as much now.

**Clare** is 27, white, lesbian and lives on her own. She has had ME for a few years and has also been deaf for several years, before which she was hard of hearing. She worked in disability organizations and race relations before she became ill, and currently does voluntary work when she has the energy.

**Eleanor** is 48, white and single. A severe stroke at the age of 25 resulted in paralysis of her left side and her arm became deformed and was amputated seven years later, at her request. Her main problem is a pain syndrome which is a result of brain damage. She did clerical work for ten years before getting a degree and now does some university teaching when she is able.

**Francesca** is 41, white, lives with her two cats and developed ME a few years ago. She worked for 13 years in various jobs, including a bail hostel and church community work, before studying theology and then disability studies. She currently receives disability benefits but is hoping to develop work in university teaching.

**Grace** is 36, white, lesbian and lives with her cat and sometimes a lodger. She has had rheumatoid arthritis for ten

## Biographies of the Women Interviewed

years, and has recently also had problems with colitis and an overactive thyroid. She used to work in disability arts and is now doing freelance theatre writing.

**Harriet** is 40, white and lives with her partner, teenage son and two daughters. She left school at 16 and worked in a library for many years. She was diagnosed with MS when she was 37, although doctors think it started as early as her late teens. She is not well enough to be able to work outside the house, as she would like.

**Helen** is 39, white and lives with her partner. As she has had diabetes since childhood, she normally finds it easy to manage, although she has had some periods of bad health in the last few years. She runs a small inner-city charity, which she enjoys but finds stressful.

**Janet** is 47, white and has lived by herself since being divorced. She has no children of her own but keeps in touch with two foster children. She has EDS and MS. She has worked in nursing and is now involved in the EDS Support Group and advising on disabled access to transport. She gets funding from a local charity which enables her to employ her own carers.

**Jasmin** is black, in her late 20s and lives with her partner. She developed post-viral fatigue a few years ago, but was lucky to get a quick diagnosis and it did not develop into ME. She was ill for a couple of years but is now much better, although she expects to have to work less hard and look after herself to avoid more serious illness.

**Jessie** is white, in her 40s, has a partner but does not live with him. She has had ME for several years. She had a stressful job in housing before she became ill, and is now very involved in co-counselling and an ME support group.

**Joyce** came to England from Jamaica in 1960 and worked as a nurse for over 20 years, before retiring due to developing diabetes. She has three grown-up sons and lives on her own. Church is a very important part of her life.

**Kabita** is 42, comes from Bangladesh and lives with her husband and three children. She developed diabetes a few years ago and has recently had a heart attack, so has given up one of her two part-time jobs (community work and university teaching). She finds working and looking after a family leaves her little opportunity to look after her own health.

**Lesley** is 33, white and lives on her own. She has radiotherapy injuries as a result of treatment for cervical cancer six years ago, has had a colostomy, urostomy and frequent surgery and hospital stays. She used to work in the civil service and was active in her trade union; she now puts her energy into a campaigning and support group for women with radiotherapy injuries.

**Maggie** is 35, white and lives with her husband and son. She developed a severely underactive thyroid following the birth of her son when she was 32, and it wasn't until two years after starting treatment with thyroxin that she felt 'back to normal' physically and mentally. However she has subsequently experienced two miscarriages and has yet to discover if and how her illness is involved.

**Marlene** is white and a 64-year-old widow who lives on her own. She used to teach but retired 15 years ago because of her rheumatoid arthritis. She is now involved in disabled people's groups and does a lot of art and craft. She is able to control her arthritis effectively through diet and tries to manage without taking a lot of painkillers.

**Mary** was born in 1948 in a rural town in Scotland. She developed ankylosing spondylitis in childhood, although it was not diagnosed until her early 20s. She has two grown-up children and lives with her second husband. She is involved with a disabled people's advice and counselling group and in amateur drama and music. She is also a Justice of the Peace.

**Maureen** is 21, black and lives on her own, but spends time with her family who live nearby. She has had epilepsy since early childhood and recently has had problems with frequent fits (which her medication is failing to prevent). She would like to work with disabled children but has not been able to get a job, so currently lives on disability benefits.

## Biographies of the Women Interviewed

**Paris** is 29, has a boyfriend but does not live with him. Her parents are Nigerian and she is a residential social worker. She has sickle-cell anaemia, which caused her few problems in childhood, but she has had frequent crises during her 20s. Her work is very important to her, as are her relationship, house and friends.

**Patricia** is 44, white and lives with her husband, teenage son and young daughter. She used to work as a paediatric nurse and now does child minding to supplement her husband's wage. She is involved with her local church, but her back problems and her fibromyalgia (which developed several years ago) make her too tired to do more work in the community as she would like.

**Rachel** is 67, white and lives with her husband who is retired. She has two grown-up sons and four grandchildren. She has had rheumatoid arthritis for over 30 years, which restricts her mobility and causes her a lot of pain. She used to be active in the Labour Party and Campaign for Nuclear Disarmament and enjoyed travelling and gardening. She finds it frustrating now that she cannot do as much.

**Sade** is 35 and lives with her parents, who come from Nigeria. She developed lupus several years ago, although it took a long time to be diagnosed. At the time of the interview she was working as a nurse, but since then has had a period of very bad health. She misses being able to go out in the evening and to travel as much as she used to.

**Sandra** is 48, white and lives with two of her five children; the other three are now grown up. She is divorced and hasn't worked outside the home since she married. She suffers from hypertension and also developed agoraphobia 19 years ago, which is getting better, but still means she spends almost all her time in the house.

**Shirley** is 48, white and lives with her husband. She was a health visitor for 14 years, until she became ill and was diagnosed as having lupus. She looks after the house and two pets, sometimes helps her husband with his antique dealing, and would like to write a novel.

**Tracey** is 24, white and developed diabetes as a baby. She lives on her own. She has recently been studying and working part time as a cashier in a supermarket, and enjoys pop music a lot. She would like to get her health better, study more, and get a better place to live.

# Glossary of Illnesses and Medical Conditions

**Arthritis and Rheumatic Diseases**: there are 200 rheumatic diseases which cause aches and pains in bones, muscles, joints, or tissues surrounding the joints; these include arthritis, which particularly attacks joints. Three women in this book have rheumatoid arthritis and have varying degrees of mobility, pain and deterioration in their hips, knees, neck or other joints. One woman has ankylosing spondylitis, which is one of the arthritis-related viruses, another has fibromyalgia, a rheumatic condition causing muscular pain and weakness.

**Asthma**: this condition affects almost eight million people in Britain and is on the increase, especially in children. There is a strong link between levels of asthma and air pollution, but the disease can also be inherited and is triggered by many different things, including stress, pollen, animals, cigarette smoke, house dust, mites, dairy products and other foods. During an attack the airways narrow, making it difficult to breathe. Some people have only mild symptoms but an attack can easily be fatal.

**Cancer**: coming in many different forms, some types of cancer respond fairly well to treatment and others are quickly fatal. The women interviewed in this book have had breast cancer and cervical cancer, both currently on the increase and attributed to various different causes. In Britain, breast cancer is the commonest fatal cancer in women and the most common cause of death in women aged between 35 and 54. As with most cancers, treatment such as chemotherapy or radiotherapy may be as painful or disabling as the disease itself. Some women have suffered severe effects from radiotherapy, such as paralysis in one arm and extreme breathlessness (after treatment for breast cancer), and damage to organs in the pelvic area (after treatment for cervical cancer), causing extreme pain, inability to digest food and inability to have sexual intercourse.

**Colitis**: an inflammation of the colon. Ulcerative colitis involves ulceration, considerable pain and the nonfunctioning of the bowel. Conventional medicine offers treatment with steroids or eventually surgery to remove part of or all of the colon. Like some other conditions related to the digestive system, colitis may be treated effectively through diet.

**Diabetes**: this is when you don't have enough of the hormone insulin in your body to convert glucose into energy. It is treated either with a strict diet alone, or diet together with either tablets or insulin injections. Some people stay very healthy with diabetes, but it can make you very tired if not well-controlled and there are long-term problems with eyesight, feet, kidneys and heart disease.

**EDS (Ehlers-Danlos Syndrome)**: EDS is an inherited connective tissue (collagen) disorder involving abnormalities of the skin, ligaments and blood vessels. Symptoms include very mobile joints (which dislocate easily), very elastic and fragile skin, a tendency to bruise easily and wounds that do not heal. People with EDS may have joint pain and a variety of other complications, but perhaps the most serious problems arise from the rarity of the disease, which means that doctors may mistreat or fail to diagnose patients.

**Epilepsy**: the second most common neurological condition after migraine, epilepsy can affect people of any age, but is especially common in younger people. Its cause is often unknown. A seizure or fit results from a temporary excess of electrical activity in the brain and can involve a variety of symptoms, from a brief 'blank' spell or muscle spasms to a complete loss of consciousness and convulsions. Medication can control the condition, although it may also have side effects such as weight gain. Some people go for years at a

## Glossary of Illnesses and Medical Conditions

time without having attacks, while others have them frequently. People with epilepsy may have to take care to avoid excessive alcohol, bright or flashing lights, stress or overexertion, all of which can trigger fits.

**Heart Disease, Hypertension and Stroke**: heart disease and strokes are second only to cancer as the most common cause of premature death in women in Britain. Two women in this book have had heart attacks (both are also diabetic), one is in her 30s and the other in her 40s. Hypertension is another term for high blood pressure, which is one of the causes of a stroke and is particularly common in black women. All these problems relating to the circulation of blood around the body are affected by many different factors, including diet, heredity, smoking and exercise. Symptoms of heart disease include pains in the chest and legs, breathlessness and faintness. Symptoms of high blood pressure include headaches, dizziness and fainting spells, but many people have no obvious symptoms.

**HIV (Human Immunodeficiency Virus)**: this is the virus thought to cause AIDS (acquired immunity deficiency syndrome). Since AIDS has only been around for a relatively short time, it is not known how long a person can live with HIV before developing AIDS, or indeed whether everyone who is HIV positive will develop AIDS. HIV weakens the immune system so that the body is vulnerable to many types of infection. Since there is no cure, a diagnosis of being HIV positive is terrifying, but it appears that people can stay healthy for longer by having a healthy diet and lifestyle.

**Lupus (Systemic Lupus Erythmatosus or SLE)**: an autoimmune disease which causes the body's immune system to attack various different organs. It is difficult to diagnose because of the range of different symptoms, and the effects can vary from mild skin problems to joint pain and serious kidney and heart disease. It affects women far more than men, and black women more than white.

**ME (Myalgic Encephalomyelitis)**: a fairly recently discovered illness, ME results from infection by a virus that stays in the cells and central nervous system because the body's immune system has failed to fight it off effectively. Varied symptoms include extreme muscle and general fatigue, sore muscles, memory and concentration loss and bowel problems. Since some doctors still do not believe in it, diagnosis can be problematic. Some people recover after a few years but others steadily deteriorate and appear never to recover.

**MS (Multiple Sclerosis)**: a disease of the central nervous system which affects more women than men. Some people live quite healthily with it for a long time, with only mild symptoms and long periods of remission, while others deteriorate very rapidly. Symptoms are very variable between individuals, but can include eyesight problems, digestive problems, loss of sensation, weakness or clumsiness and, very commonly, extreme fatigue.

**Sickle-Cell Anaemia**: an inherited blood disorder which affects people of Afro-Caribbean descent. In a sickle-cell 'crisis' the red blood cells in the body turn to the shape of a sickle moon (hence the name) and cannot move through the veins properly, causing agonizing pain all over the body. People may go for many years feeling perfectly well with it, but tiredness, stress, dehydration or illness can provoke a crisis which can be fatal if not treated properly.

**Spina Bifida**: this is caused by a defect in the neural tube – which forms the brain and spinal column – while the embryo is developing in the womb. Many people are born with some form of spina bifida, but its severity varies widely. Some children do not survive long after birth or have to undergo extensive surgery, while other people experience almost no effects at all. Others still may deteriorate gradually during adulthood, eventually experiencing considerable disability and pain.

**Thyroid Disease**: the thyroid gland produces hormones which regulate the body's metabolism and it can become overactive or underactive (so, for example, producing symptoms such as a very quick heart rate and diarrhoea or a sluggish heart rate and constipation respectively). An underactive thyroid can be treated by taking thyroxin (the missing

## Glossary of Illnesses and Medical Conditions

hormone) daily, but an overactive thyroid is often treated by getting rid of part of the thyroid gland with surgery or radioactivity, either of which is likely to lead to an underactive thyroid.

There are charities or support groups dealing with all these illnesses and many others. If you need more information or advice, you may be able to get contact addresses by asking a nurse or doctor. Otherwise look in the phone directory and library or contact your local Community Health Council, Well Woman clinic, Citizens Advice Bureau, Council for Voluntary Service or various advertized patient information services.

# Index

Abortion, termination 130, 131
Abuse, sexual (*see also* Sexual harassment) 24, 39–40, 42, 107–8, 129, 189–90
  from partners (*see also* Violence) 69–70
Acceptance 42, 43–6
Access, to buildings, housing 54, 60, 69–70, 136
  as barrier to social life 82–3
Action for Victims of Medical Accidents 175
Adoption, fostering 131–2, 135–6
Advertising, charities 3
  television 21
Advice *see* Information
Age, growing older, older women 17, 46, 65, 95, 161–2, 180
Agoraphobia 5, 31
Alcott, Louisa 94
AIDS (*see also* HIV) 5, 16, 74, 131, 163–4, 165, 188, 194, 196
Alcoholism 5
Anger 43, 45
Ankylosing spondylitis 5, 66, 178, 187
Anorexia 5
Anxiety 34–5
  anxiety attacks 168
Arthritis 5, 19, 20, 30, 35, 43, 46, 57, 64, 90–91, 111, 148, 149, 163, 169, 180, 185
Assertion, assertiveness 173–4
Asthma 5, 74, 169

Benefits, Benefits System 43, 51, 60, 67, 70, 91, 152
Black women, Black people 18, 144, 164, 205
  disbelief by medical profession 180–81
  lack of appropriate information 166
Blame and responsibility 183–209
  victim-blaming, blaming the powerless 191–6
Bodies and body image, 19–21, 101
  idealized body 19, 193
  weight, control 35–6
  weight, medical prejudices about 144, 181
British Diabetic Association (BDA) 1, 3
British Medical Association (BMA) 148

Caesarean section 131
Cancer (*see also* Mastectomy, Radiotherapy) 5, 14, 38, 89, 90, 105–6, 115, 140–42, 151, 162, 180, 186, 188, 191–2, 194, 201, 203, 209
Caring, for others 66, 68–9, 136
  men and caring 114–16, 119–20
  women and caring 114–17
Causes of illness 183–4, 191, 199
Cerebral palsy 129
Changes, in our abilities/needs 78–9

# Index

difficulties for our partners 120–21
difficulties for families 121
Charities 3, 175, 196
Childbirth, effect on sex 107
Childhood, illness/disability in 3, 25–9
Childhood trauma (*see also* Abuse) 184, 190
Children (*see also* Motherhood) 101, 126–7, 129–37
  as reason for living 137
  attitudes to disability 76
  being taken into care 132
  changes in adult/child relationship 134
  helping with housework, as carers 134–5
Chloroquine 36, 78
Choice, lack of in medical treatment 146
Class, family background, differences in relationships 113–14
Closed in, cut off from others 87
Cole, Juanita 180, 208
Colleagues at work 55–6, 92
Colostomy 14, 85, 105
Compensation, making complaints about health care, legal action 141, 146–7, 175
Complementary medicine/therapies 37, 149–50, 199–201
  lack of information on 166
Community, 'care in the community' 95
  lack of community spirit 95
Community Health Councils 175–6
Community Health workers 162
Confidence, loss of 36, 49–50, 108
Conflicting explanations for illness 184–90
Consent, informed 147
Contagion, contamination, fear of 15, 73–4
Contraception, control of reproduction 129, 131, 144

Contraceptive pill 189, 192
Control, loss of 33–7, 81–2
  over health 192–3, 201
Cure 43, 44–5
Curiosity, fascination with disability 75–7
Cystic fibrosis 198

Deadly Experiments 6
Deafness 79, 126
Death, bereavement 88
  fear of, coming to terms with 35, 38–44, 89, 115, 192, 209
  images of 22
Denial, disbelief, doubt 12, 13, 28–9, 55, 92, 115
  from medical profession 148, 176–82, 188, 195
  within family 123
Dependence/independence 101, 123–4, 128
  in relationship with doctors 143–8
  women seen as dependent 112–13, 129–30
Depo Provera 129
Depression 5, 30
Diabetes 1, 5, 9, 10, 25, 27, 36, 37, 57, 58, 59, 74, 81, 82, 105, 115, 125, 126–8, 132, 136–7, 149, 165, 167, 169, 170, 173, 185, 196, 198, 203, 207
Diagnosis 28, 39, 176–7, 181–2, 195
Diet (*see also* Food), 35, 146, 149–50, 167
Difference 4, 11–12
  different concerns from healthy people 10, 88
Disabled people's movement 2–3, 54, 65, 201–5
Dislocation, and separation from normal world 10–11
Doctors *see* Medical Profession
Donne, John 209

Economic stresses, recession, poverty 51, 95
Eczema 30

EDS (Ehlers Danlos Syndrome) 28, 164–5, 169, 185
Education 25–6, 27
  access to children's school 136
Employers 51, 55, 56, 57–9, 67
Employment *see* Work
Endometriosis 168
Energy levels, lower than other people's 83–4, 118–19
Environment, pollution 184, 191, 193
Epilepsy 5, 10, 20, 25, 53, 57, 65, 67, 73, 110, 167, 185
Equal opportunities 51, 57
Equipment, medical, walking aids 74, 77–8
Eugenics, eugenist views 144

Family/families (*see also* Childhood) 86, 89, 97, 101–39
  wider family 127
  having no family 128–9
Fear, other people's, of contagion 15
  of death/desertion 89, 115, 192
  of difference/disability 74–5, 76
Fear, our own, of being alone 39
  of death 38–44, 192, 209
  of disability or illness in our children 132–3, 136
  of further illness 154
  of losing job 59
  of relationships 110
Feminine identity 22–3
  images of womanhood and femininity (*see also* Body image, Sexuality) 7, 21, 101–2
Feminism, feminists 117, 201–205
Fenton Thomas, Paula 166
Fibromyalgia 5
Finger, Anne 3, 191
Fits (*see also* Epilepsy) 81, 82
Food (*see also* Diet) 126
  as restriction on social life 85
Freedom, loss of 33–7
Friendship(s), friends 72, 84, 86, 88–91, 94
  abusive, rejection by 92, 98
  helpful, supportive 96–9
  made through becoming disabled 99
Frustration, at low energy levels 62
Full-time work 49, 60, 64

Genetic causes of disease 184–5, 191, 197–9
Gender, in employment *see* Women's work/employment
Generations, different ideas about health 124, 126
Girlfriends, friends and partners 90, 116–17
GP (General Practitioner) 143, 145, 148, 155, 157
Gratitude, having to be grateful 93–4
  towards medical profession 146–7, 156–7
Guilt, in relationships/families 119–21, 122–3, 137

Health information *see* Information
Health Service (*see also* Medical profession) 5–7, 55, 68, 140–82, 143, 146, 147, 160, 195
  cuts, changes in 95, 141, 158–9, 162, 198–9, 200
  good experiences of 155–60
  hierarchies, structure of, barriers to good care 171–2
  women as patients of 143–4, 150
Heart disease, heart attacks 5, 169, 177
Help, need for, requesting, getting what we need 79, 80, 81, 93, 97
Hereditary illness *see* Genetic causes of disease
High blood pressure *see* hypertension
HIV (*see also* AIDS) 5, 16, 37, 38, 39, 60, 69, 88, 103, 159, 163, 165, 188, 194
Holistic approach 199–201
  lack of within conventional

# Index

medicine 168
Hospitality, helping others, restrictions on 87
Housework 41, 61, 63, 66, 68, 116, 119–20
Human insulin *see* Insulin
Hypertension, high blood pressure 5, 31
Hysterectomy 140, 150

Iatrogenesis 150
Identity 9–47, 16–18, 44–7, 63, 65–6
  feminine 22–3
  lesbian 18, 23
Income support *see* Benefits
Independence *see* Dependence
Information, about health 155–6
  advantages of being well-informed 173–4
  changes in medical advice/information 170–71
  conflicting, and conflicting treatment 167, 168–70
  problems with, lack of 160–67
Inspiration, sick people as 94
Insulin 36, 77, 138
Invisibility (*see also* Visibility) 9–47, 79–80
Invisible illnesses and symptoms 12–19
Invisible women 12–19
Isolation 9–12, 9–47
  and feelings of desertion by doctors 151–54
IVF (in vitro fertilization) 168

Jealousy 90–92
John, Alison 129

Lesbian identity 18, 23
Lesbian relationships 104, 116
Lesbians, as hidden group, 'passing as normal' 15, 77
  excluded from feminist movement 205
Leisure 64–5
Liberation 38–9
Lorde, Audre 12, 89, 106, 166, 201

Lupus (systemic lupus erythmatosus, SLE) 5, 55, 79, 163, 166, 186

Management of own illness 144–5
Mason, Micheline 130
Mastectomy 12, 45, 105–6, 120, 150, 151, 203
Maternity Alliance 129–30, 185
ME (myalgic encephalomyelitis) 5, 15, 22, 30, 40, 60, 76, 79, 126, 177, 187–9, 195–6, 203
Medical notes, access to 141
Medical profession (*see also* Health Service) 5–7, 140–82, 184, 188, 196, 202
  good experiences of 155–60
  ignorance and prejudice 163–7
Medication, medical and other equipment 72, 74, 106
Men, as carers 114–16, 119–20
  attitudes to health 23–4, 115
  attitudes to women 112–13, 114
Menstruation, menstrual cycle 19, 21, 24, 165
  hormones and women's health 178–9
Mental health/illness 5, 31, 73
  mental hospital, psychiatric wards 131, 177, 195
  women assumed to have psychosomatic illness 177–8
Mental impairment, learning disability 73, 129
Middle class women 4, 195–6
Money, income 49, 60, 70–71
  lack of, as restriction on social life 86
Morrison, Kathleen 6
Motherhood, and disabled women, attitudes towards 129–31
  medical advice on pregnancy 130–31
MS (multiple sclerosis) 15, 79, 124, 129, 169, 178

National Health Service *see* Health Service
Needs, at work 56–8

Normality 15, 21, 48
Nursing (as profession) 55–6

Older women *see* Age
Other people 9, 72–99

Pain 13–14, 29–32, 63, 79, 137
   disbelief of pain by health workers (*see also* Black people, Racism) 148, 164, 180–81, 182, 180–81
   in sickle-cell anaemia 164, 180
Parents 94, 121–26
   fear, blaming us for ill-health 125
Partner(s), attitudes of 42, 90, 92, 94, 138–9
   fears about caring 112–15
   husband(s), boyfriend(s) 77, 84, 93, 111, 114
   not having a partner 110, 111
   woman partner(s) 90, 116
Part-time work 49, 61
*Past Due* 3
Patients Association 175
Penicillin 125
Periods *see* Menstruation
Pesticides 191–2
Physical activity 21, 118–19
Physical access *see* Access
Positive changes, discoveries 39–42, 64, 96
Positive thinking 201
Positively Women 39, 103, 159, 163
Poverty 68, 70–71, 95, 192–4, 206
Pressures on other people (*see also* Economic stresses, Poverty), in employment 56
 in society 95
Pregnancy 130–31, 132, 133, 185, 203
Prostheses 106, 204
Puerperal psychosis 131

Race, racism, racist attitudes (*see also* Black women) 27, 164, 180–81
Radiation, nuclear 6
Radiotherapy, radiotherapy injuries 14, 36, 102, 116, 133, 140–42, 147, 169, 171, 183, 184
RAGE (Radiotherapy Action Group Exposure) 141, 203
Relationships, abusive *see* Abuse, Violence
   general with other people 72–99
   heterosexual, married 101, 107, 109
   inequality in 107, 117–20
   lesbian 104, 116–17
   loss of 92
   new, potential 109–10
   with friends *see* Friendship
   with medical profession 143–82
   with other disabled people 99, 118
Religious faith 44
Research, medical experiments 6, 141, 186, 196
Responsibility, individual 184, 193
Responsibility, for others *see* Caring Rheumatic illnesses 177
Rights, to health care, income 70–71
Role, women's (*see also* Identity) 68, 116

Sciatica 153
Screening, for cancer 140, 142
 in pregnancy 132
Self-esteem/self-worth 123, 154, 202
   feeling second rate/put down 72, 84, 87
Self-help/support groups, support from others with same illness 88, 115, 120, 151, 175, 202–5
Self-image 63
Sex 102–5, 109
   for HIV-positive women 103
   heterosexual 102–4
   in lesbian relationships 104
Sexual abuse *see* Abuse
Sexual harassment 24
Sexuality (*see also* Body image,

# Index

Femininity)
disabled women 24, 102
feeling non-sexual, unattractive, not in control of body 101, 105–7, 109
loss of desire for sex 102
lesbian 77, 104
male attitudes to female sexuality, to disabled women 102–3, 112–13
male 194
Shange, Ntozake, 18
Sick leave 50, 51, 59
Sickle-cell anaemia 5, 26, 30, 44, 72, 75, 79, 91, 109–10, 121, 133, 164, 180, 184–5, 198
Sister(s) 83, 91, 122
SLE *see* Lupus
Social contact, social life 48–9, 72, 81
restrictions on 82–4, 86
Social security *see* Benefits
Social services 69, 71, 95
*Spell # 7* 18
Spina bifida 5, 28, 43, 153, 185
Steroids 167
Stigma 73, 74, 77, 199
Stress 184, 186, 187–8, 189, 193
Stroke 42, 79, 153
Studying 52–3

T-cell count 60
*The Cancer Journals* 12, 89, 106, 166
Thyroid disease, underactivethyroid 5, 121, 133, 178, 182
Thyroxin 168
Time, for self 40
lack of in medical care 171–2
Tiredness, fatigue, exhaustion 13, 31–2, 56, 57, 86

as barrier to social life 82–4
Travel/Transport 33–4

Unpredictability, uncertainty (*see also* Changes) 31–2, 61–2, 86
Urostomy 14

Variation, in our abilities *see* Changes
of severity within same illness 79
Violence, images of 22
in family 28, 69–70
Visibility 72–8, 75, 77, 79–80
Viruses 186–7
Voluntary sector 57
Voluntary work 49, 63–4, 65, 67

Walking, ability to walk 33, 78, 83–4
Well Women Clinics 175
Wheelchairs *see* Equipment
wheelchair users, prejudice towards 15, 77, 78
wheelchair, changes/choice about using 77, 78
Women, defined in contrast to men 19–20, 22–4
male attitudes towards 112–13
Work 48–71
employment 51, 54
women's work/employment 53–4, 70
women's work in home (*see also* Roles) 68–9, 95, 116
Working class women 17, 27, 95, 144, 181, 195, 205
disbelief by medical profession 180–82
Women's health, attitudes towards 23–4